BRAIN CHANGE
An Understanding of Addiction

JOHN E. "JACK" DALEY

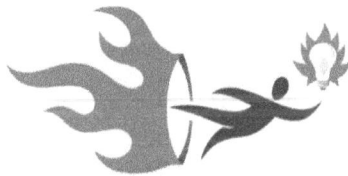

Burning Bulb
PUBLISHING

Brain Change: An Understanding of Addiction
By **John E. "Jack" Daley**

Burning Bulb Publishing
P.O. Box 4721
Bridgeport, WV 26330-4721
United States of America
www.BurningBulbPublishing.com

Cover designed by Gary Lee Vincent

First Edition.

Paperback Edition ISBN: 978-1-964172-34-7

FOREWORD

Welcome. The text you are about to read results from 35 years of treating alcoholics, addicts, their families, employers, and friends, as well as those who loved them, hated them, arrested them, shed tears over them, and even married them. You see, chances are good that if you chose to read this, your life has been impacted by an addiction – either your own or that of someone you care about. No one chooses to suffer from an addiction, yet they are related to enough medical problems to constitute the #1 health issue in the nation.

Having dedicated much of my life to addiction care, I witnessed countless changes in the treatment of those affected, and sometimes destroyed, by drugs and alcohol. Despite this, I found almost no one – not among medical professionals, drug counselors, law enforcement, psychologists nor men of the cloth who could agree on a *simple, uniform definition of addiction.*

Without a stable understanding of addictions, treatment is ineffective. Addictions affect one of every four Americans. The damage to health, careers and families is said to touch virtually all of us at some time during our lives. Yet, if the best minds cannot agree on the causes of addiction, the measures of success or what constitutes recovery, treatment will continue to falter.

Brain Change: An Understanding of Addiction is not another text parroting the ideas of others. It expands upon current definitions of addiction uniting medical, mental health, societal and behavioral functioning. The reader will examine the effects of drugs and alcohol seeing how their use impacts issues from neurology to family values. Using personal vignettes, the book takes an uncompromising look at addictions from early onset through their inevitable and often tragic conclusions. Ultimately, ***Brain Change*** is for anyone whose life is touched by addiction.

The author and publisher have neither liability nor responsibility to any person or organization regarding injury, loss or damage caused by information contained in this book. I have added changes to the definitions and facts about addiction found in most textbooks. These changes, although minor, are far from insignificant and every effort has been made to ensure accuracy. ***Brain Change*** expands upon current definitions, giving the reader an understanding of addiction's effects upon physical and mental health as well as upon the values and chemical makeup of those who become addicted. The reader will come away with expanded awareness of what constitutes addiction and what it takes to overcome one.

DEDICATION

Brain Change: An Understanding of Addiction examines most addictions, covering standard categories of drugs and modes of drug use. From early-stage addicts through terminal users, young through elderly, high achievers to those barely literate, this book examines those affected by commonly abused drugs, explaining their effects upon individuals, families, and our society.

There are many who crossed my life over the years whom I wish to thank. Among these are medical professionals, colleagues, supervisors, and friends. Of course, the greatest impact was from clients. I mention early in this book that my clients were some of the finest people I had ever met – keeping in mind that many were thieves, killers, con artists, and some frightening people. But the majority were different when they found recovery. I thank all of you and I hope the knowledge shared in this book helps build a new generation of those who understand and treat addictions.

Brain Change is dedicated to the toughest, most non-compliant, and frustrating people I have ever met: my clients – for your recoveries are truly a miracle. Through your struggles, pain, successes, and failures, you have demonstrated strength to overcome adversities that I could only imagine in my worst nightmares. With all my heart, I thank you.

TABLE OF CONTENTS

INTRODUCTION

It was sometime in mid-1985, and I was having coffee with my supervising psychiatrist when a colleague stuck her head in the doorway to tell me that one of my patients had just died. The late Mr. Parnell was a nice old man who just could not see the sense of not drinking, no matter how much his liver cried foul. As a drug and alcohol counselor, my job was to try to find the key to motivating people like Mr. Parnell and halt their march to oblivion. The response to my colleague was something like, "Yes, it's too bad, but that's life." I then continued my chat with the doctor about the previous night's ball game.

Dr. K. is a kind, gentle man with a desire to make all his patients read Ayn Rand's _Atlas Shrugged_. I always found that kind of unusual, but he was a great psychiatrist – and his patients loved him. This day though, he took offense at my seeming lack of compassion. His eyes widened and he stared at me over his glasses, assuming his "supervisor" persona, informing me that in his 10 years of practice he had lost twelve patients and always took it very hard. He added that he was surprised at my rather cavalier attitude toward a patient's death. While I had no intention of trying to shock the good doctor, I reminded him that my area of treatment was addictions. Over a similar 10-year period I had seen close to 100 die from alcohol or drug use. He paused for a long moment and said, "I suppose you get used to it."

No, you don't Doc. Believe me. You never get used to it.

No one ever planned on being an alcoholic or an addict. "Johnny, what do you want to be when you grow up? A fireman, a truck driver?"

"I want to be a junkie like my dad."

It does not work that way. No one…not you, not me nor anyone who ever picked up a drink, a joint or a pill, or snorted a powder, or spiked a needle thought that he or she was going to become addicted.

Perhaps it starts with that adolescent feeling of immortality that says, "It'll never happen to me." But it happens to millions. Addictions, when you consider all of them and their related afflictions, constitute the #1 health problem in the country – and not one person ever planned on it happening to them.

At the same time, treating addictions is not high on the list of occupations found in the high school guidance office. Working with addicts in any stage of recovery can be akin to its own untreatable form of mental illness. As a group, addictions counselors are looked down on by medical staff, fellow mental health providers and the legal profession. It is an occupation rife with incompetent do-gooders and often equally incompetent professionals. It is only over the past few decades that things have improved with ongoing professional standards and proper supervision. The pay in addiction treatment has improved, but most of those providing care work multiple jobs to pay the bills. The clients, even when clean and sober, are often the most non-compliant, demanding people on earth. Many have personality disorders resulting from abuse and neglect and some are dangerously crazy. (It is quite an experience to find out that the person sitting alone with you in a sound-proof office has been controlling his homicidal impulses for the past few years with illicit drugs and is now hearing voices that make him very suspicious of you…but more about those adventures later.) Addicts often lie to you for the sake of doing it – and sometimes because they do not know the difference between lies and the truth.

So why does anyone do this for a living when the night shift at a fast-food-joint pays almost as well? To paraphrase the words of experts in addiction studies, "…you become addicted to addicts." That explains much of it, for the work has intrinsic rewards found only in helping the hopeless and occasionally witnessing some real miracles. Addiction treatment is not just a job, it is a calling – one replete with enough aggravation for ten lifetimes, but enough rewards for a thousand. Sorry if that statement sounds preachy. Although the work can be very rewarding, working with addicts is a lot of hard and sometimes dangerous work.

But that does not explain why I, or anyone else, enters this field. Most who do so start out with a little "practical experience," often having messed up their own lives with alcohol or drugs. By age 26, I had already lost one career, was back living with my parents, and dating women who drank like me. That last quality also meant that most of them were not exactly someone I was taking home to meet Mom.

Another unnerving issue was that my best friend in high school was now in Washington D.C. working for a politician on a highly publicized committee and showing up on TV regularly. He was making history while I was working second shift in a mill making grinding wheels. At some point I realized that I was never going to be the person I wanted to be unless I changed my lifestyle. So, I did. I will always add a sincere "Thanks" to the self-help groups that made it so much easier.

With recovery comes a need to make positive changes. Feeling better about oneself, coupled with wanting to share your experience with others who have the same problem, makes many become instant do-gooders. A career in addiction treatment often starts there. But the desire to help others will not get the job done properly. Skills, education, tough supervision, and a willingness to learn from your mistakes makes working in addictions as challenging as it is fascinating. You might even do some good along the way.

It is my hope that this book will provide future counselors, social workers, medical staff, law enforcement, and those in recovery with a realistic understanding of addictions and their treatments. The vignettes are as true to fact as my memory, clouded by time and circumstances, can recall. All names and major identifying details have been changed to protect confidentiality. I never recorded a session and only quoted clients in my clinical notes when necessary. As a result, any subsequent quotations are only as accurate as my recall allows them to be. The words of clients, like the incidents around them, have softened my feelings for even the most difficult and resistant people. For them, their histories, struggles, successes, and losses provide a look at a way of life unimagined by those who have never struggled with addictions.

SECTION I

ADDICTS:
ALL SHAPES AND SIZES

CHAPTER 1
WHY DO WE DO THIS?

The first person I saw die from an addiction was Patrick, a 47-year-old defrocked Catholic priest. He died of liver failure after a lifetime of addiction to alcohol that cost him his calling, his friends, his self-respect, his health, and finally, his life. Patrick had no history of mistreating others nor any behavioral issues other than he drank too much. He had multiple attempts at treatment but could never stop drinking for any extended period. Patrick was admitted to our detoxification unit after going into *delirium tremens* when he tried to stop drinking on his own. Delirium tremens (*def.*) is *an acute form of withdrawal from alcohol. The "D.T's" come in stages lasting up to two weeks with extreme agitation, confusion and terrifying hallucinations. There is severe anxiety, paranoia and delusions accompanied by violent tremors and perspiration that can soak through bedding.* A teacher at a private high school prior to his admission, Patrick was liked by students and staff alike. There was never any question about his skills nor his character. His friends and colleagues respected his intellect and his talent. He was simply addicted to alcohol.

This book takes a hard look at many like Patrick who suffer from some form of addiction, the #1 health problem in the nation. Addiction is related to one of every four deaths in America, yet every treatment discipline has its own definition. Addiction is seen as a mental health problem, a moral weakness, a medical complication, a lack of willpower and a major social issue. With little effort I found multiple definitions for addiction depending upon which discipline was being followed. It must be noted that no other disease, no other medical problem comes with such a confusing array of definitions. Among these:

(1.) Addiction is regularly performed attempts at pleasurable stimulation resulting in a progressive pattern of use, often with mild to extreme craving upon cessation of use. (It features) compulsive, relapsing and often uncontrolled dependence on a habit, substance, or practice to such a degree that cessation causes emotional, mental, or physiologic reactions. (Mosby's Medical, Nursing and Allied Health Dictionary) 4th Ed., 1994

(2.) (Addiction is) physical or psychological, or both, dependence on a substance, esp. alcohol or drugs, with use of increasing amounts. (Taber's cyclopedic Medical Dictionary) 15th edition

(3.) The essential feature of a substance abuse disorder (addiction) is a cluster of cognitive, behavioral, and physiological symptoms indicating that the individual continues using the substance despite significant substance-related problems. (Diagnostic and Statistical Manual of Mental Disorders, Fifth Edition, or DSM-5, Substance abuse disorders, features.)

(4.) Addiction is any repeated behavior, substance-related or not, in which a person feels compelled to persist, regardless of its negative impact on his life and the lives of others. (In the Realm of Hungry Ghosts) Gabor Mate' M.D.

(5.) The state of being addicted esp. to a habit-forming drug, to such an extent that cessation causes severe trauma. (The Random House College Dictionary, Unabridged Ed., 1973)

(6.) Addiction is a neuropsychological disorder characterized by a persistent and intense urge to use a drug or engage in behavior that produces natural reward, despite substantial harm or other negative consequences. (Wikipedia)

(7.) Addiction is a treatable chronic medical disease involving complex interactions among brain circuits, genetics, the environment, and an individual's life experiences. (Wikipedia)

(8.) Addictions develop from a combination of choice, and additional factors, including genetics, trauma history, related mental health issues such as depression and anxiety, and personal losses or conflicts. Addictions are affected by a person's culture and environment and over time, the person loses his ability to choose whether or not to use. (American Society of Addiction Medicine)

These definitions are similar - yet all are different. Each discipline, whether it be medicine, mental health, legal, religious or some variation, defines addiction from their own perspective while excluding those that differ. The treatment provider must ultimately understand that the person sitting in front of him, no matter how their symptoms manifest, is an individual whose combination of symptoms may be found in no others.

My time with Patrick was brief as I held his hand while he trembled and perspired profusely. Unable to say much, he knew he was very ill. His skin was orange and the whites of his eyes were deep yellow rimmed in red. He was bloated around the middle, a condition called *ascites, (def.) an abnormal buildup of fluid in the abdominal cavity often found with acute liver failure.* I do not know if he was aware he was dying, but his eyes stared across the room in abject terror. One of the difficulties of treating someone in D.T.'s is that the medications used to reduce withdrawal symptoms cannot be broken down by the liver because the organ is so damaged. The medications themselves then become toxic. Subsequently, if the withdrawal does not get you, the medications will. Patrick died a few days after admission.

As Patrick's counselor, it was my job to contact his employer, the school principal, of his death. The principal made the usual expressions of shock and sadness and told me what a great teacher he was and how staff and kids alike thought the world of him. Then he added something I was to hear too often. "We all knew he had a problem...but he was such a great guy. No one knew what to do. We didn't want to endanger his job." So, they did nothing and watched him drink himself to death. At least they did not endanger his job.

Later, my supervisor, a crusty ex-merchant seaman, pointed out that Patrick, once a priest and "man of God," died because "Even

God couldn't keep him sober. God is like the guy in the tool crib…He hands out the tools, but if you don't use them, he won't fix things for you." The analogy is crude, but effective.

Alcohol and drug dependence are generational problems. It is not unusual to have second, third, and even fourth-generation alcoholics or addicts in treatment. There are hereditary factors that we will look at later, but in the "nature vs. nurture" debate, it is a fact that children grow up influenced by the behaviors, attitudes, and beliefs of their parents. *The most powerful force parents give their children is the power of their own example…and if that example is to escape through chemicals, then this is the behavior their children will see as normal.* A child may not like a parent's drinking or drug use, but that child will likely learn to handle life with chemicals – just like Mom or Dad. It is unusual to meet an addict of any kind who did not grow up in a family where people escaped, relaxed or rewarded themselves with alcohol, drugs or some other unhealthy habit. Coupled with this, the children of addicts often grow up *parentified, (def.) assuming responsibilities for themselves and younger siblings that are far beyond their years.* Subsequently, they get blamed and scapegoated for family problems caused by parents who can barely care for themselves properly, let alone their children. These children develop a distorted self-image and grow up hurt and angry. They act out toward others or overcompensate with unhealthy behaviors and by seeking solace the way they learned it from their parents – through chemicals. As I sat each day with sick, addicted, and mentally ill clients, I often wondered where their lives would have taken them had circumstances steered them away from addiction.

THE GHETTO PHILOSOPHER

Manny looked like an addict. From the first day he walked into my office, his gaunt physique, sallow complexion and overall unkempt appearance gave away his battle with drugs. Addicts do not like to stand out. Manny could not hide it though. It was a gift from his parents.

Manny was a half-Irish, half-Puerto Rican kid born in a Bronx tenement. As a child, he and his four siblings moved from one bad neighborhood to another before his family relocated to the projects of Worcester, Massachusetts. They settled in a part of the city called Great Brook Valley which, during the 1980's, was the epicenter for drug dependence in the city. I met Manny in 1983 when "The Valley" was a classic city ghetto, a public housing development whose inhabitants were kept hostage by drug dealers and gangs. Manny once told me that there are people in the Valley who never leave except to get more drugs to sell. They never get beyond the projects from birth to death. They know little and contribute less. But they make money dealing drugs. Manny would get angry as he talked about the Valley. It was as though he wanted to blame his problems on the ghetto he called home. He had been stabbed the week before I met him and was recovering from surgery to repair a damaged hand.

Manny's parents were both chronic alcoholics. One of his three sisters had a lengthy history of prostitution arrests and the other two had long ago disappeared into the foster care system. A younger brother bounced in and out of jail for a few years before finding his own recovery. Manny married a few years before I met him and his wife was a spitfire. Julia was a pretty Hispanic girl with a lot of spirit. Once, while looking for Manny, she went charging into a "shooting gallery," the back room of a store where heroin users gathered to get high together. This is the type of place the police employed a SWAT team to break into. Manny said, "You should have seen the place empty out. No one was gonna tangle with Julia."

Manny showed up in my office on orders from his probation officer. He had recently completed a jail term where he kicked his heroin habit but needed a lot of help to remain clean. Manny did well for quite a long time. He loved to talk, and despite being a 10th grade dropout, he read newspapers and magazines voraciously. For fun, during the summer "flea market" season, he would buy old physics and calculus textbooks and study them. He said that is why he liked Worcester. With ten colleges within its boundaries, he could always find old text books. Manny loved math, science and philosophy. He would often try to distract me by sharing his philosophical views rather than addressing his addiction. I did a lot of redirecting with Manny. He knew when I was getting aggravated with him and loved to make that happen. But still, he did well.

One day, Manny told me he had gotten a "gig."

"A what? I asked.

"A gig…you know, a music gig…with a group."

Now by this time I had been seeing Manny for months and had no idea he played any musical instrument. "Yeh, I found a saxophone in an abandoned building a couple of years ago. I taught myself to play it." Manny joined up with three other guys and they had a little band, playing neighborhood parties and even an occasional wedding. The kid had more natural skills than most.

Manny struggled with periodic relapses for a couple of years. One led to an overdose that nearly killed him and during another, Julia left him, taking their two young daughters with her. I feared this would send him into an endless cycle of relapses, but it proved to be the motivator for Manny to finally stay clean. Before long, he was drug-free, attending self-help and had realistic plans for the future. Oh yes, Julia took him back after a few months.

Manny got a maintenance job at a local college where one of the fringe benefits was free tuition for employees. He eventually got an Associate degree and was working on a Bachelor degree when I last saw him. As with many others, I hated to see Manny leave, but he did not need counseling any longer.

On his last visit, I asked Manny where he thought his life would have gone had he been given the opportunities in his youth that others had been given. He thought for a moment and said, "Life is the only opportunity we need. There are no guarantees other than the chance to grow beyond the mistakes of your parents. If I'd been born rich and handsome, I would have just made different mistakes, maybe worse ones, and would be somewhere else. I'm happy to be right where I am, right now."

Manny left his problems and his parental addictions behind him and developed a pretty good philosophy for life, moving beyond the scars of his childhood. Tragically, not everyone has Manny's innate ability to overcome negative parental influences. Unlike Manny, some get worse and remain victims while taking others with them.

A GOOD KID

You can be assured that "Beef" is one of the few convicted triple murderers walking the streets of a major New England city – or hopefully any other city. He did them too – and a few others, I am sure. Beef's given name was Reynold, a far more distinguished moniker. He was twice convicted of murder, once at age 15 in Alabama, for which he served 14 years, then for a double murder, which cost him 18 more years. Today, he is walking the streets a free man and, let us all hope, remaining clean and sober. Beef told me he had eight "notches" on his belt, one for each person he had killed. Addicts often like to impress others, especially men like Beef whose identity is wrapped up in his convict persona. It is likely, though, that he has at least that many murders in his history.

When I met Beef, he was in his early 50's. He was very soft-spoken and his affect was flat, betraying no emotion or pain. He was always extremely polite and took pride in his appearance and cleanliness. His attitude towards women was gracious. A tall man with a soft voice, one would never picture this man as someone with a lifetime of violent crimes.

Beef earned his stripes in a notorious New York Maximum Security prison. The men in the prison blocks or units refer to each other as "dogs." Beef was "#1 Dog." On two separate occasions, men who were in prison with Beef found it necessary to talk to me about him after seeing him in line for methadone. This was quite unusual since I never heard men talk about others they had served time with. But they both talked about how scary and "crazy" Beef was. They would never admit to being afraid of him, but it sure looked that way.

I was working in a methadone clinic in Worcester, Massachusetts, when Beef was assigned to me. I ran a weekly orientation group for clients new to the methadone program. From this group, I sometimes got to choose clients that I would work with on a weekly basis. I liked older clients and Beef was my age. He had a long history of violence and did a lot of drugs while incarcerated, dealing dope to other inmates that had been smuggled in. That, along with his intimidating behaviors, became his base of power in prison.

Beef was on parole, as were many of my clients, and was living with his mother. He was quiet, cooperative, and street-wise. And he was interesting. He told me that, above all, he did not want to go back to prison. "I like my room…I do my bit there. I watch TV and I sit on the porch. It's quiet. It's never quiet in prison."

During one of my first meetings with Beef, as part of his intake, I asked him what he did, which was his occupation. His reply was memorable. "I'm a killer. You're a counselor. Kathy (the nurse dispensing the methadone) is a nurse. I'm a killer. It's what I do. I only kill when I have to, though."

Far more than the usual assortment of burglars, shoplifters and prostitutes found in the methadone clinic, Beef provided a challenge. Dr. A., our resident psychiatrist, took me aside and told me that Beef was the most dangerous man he had ever met. "I had a serial killer when I lived in Syria. He killed 15 people," he said. "This guy is more dangerous. Be careful."

Beef got off to a rough start in life. When he was born, his mother thought he was ugly and put him in a box on top of a cupboard. A neighbor had to feed him for the first few months. It went downhill from there. His mother eventually began to feed and clothe him but her boyfriends, those who would not beat him, ignored him. He bonded with no one.

Beef could recall parts of those first years, but as is often seen with victims of repeated trauma, he blocked out many of the people and details. He could not remember all the places he had lived, although he remembered living in Alabama for a few years. He remembered eating cereal. Not just for breakfast either. Three meals a day, every day. Mom did not like cooking. He remembered little about most of the men his mother lived with, nor could he recall the birth of his sister. His first legal issues sprang up around the age of seven when he was placed in a series of foster homes for running away. He talked about being "hurt" in at least one home, but, like a lot of sex abuse victims, he could not open that door. Beef seemed genuinely relieved when I told him that at any time if he did not want to talk about something, we could "put it on the back burner" and deal with it later, perhaps never if it was too painful. I told him we would work with his drug use and leave things like abuse out of it unless he felt like handling it. He liked that, and I believe he saw it as respect, for he worked well with me.

This offers an important note for anyone providing counseling or psychotherapy: One of the worst mistakes providers make is pushing too hard and too quickly to get a client to open up about abusive, painful, or embarrassing details from their past. Clients often use defensive behavior to "shut down" and conceal the most difficult incidents in their memories. These issues can be denied or covered up for years and can be closely wrapped up in unhealthy behaviors like drug abuse. One of my long-term clients worked through a terrible history of sexual abuse by an "uncle," abuse that was denied by his mother, who made him feel responsible for it when the abuse came to light. I worked with him for two years before I dared discuss what I knew to be at the root of much of his anger and pain. *Do not ignore the issue – just know enough to not rush into discussing it. Get to know your clients before you start digging into their past. Few, if any, are willing to open up about terrible issues like abuse to someone whom they cannot yet trust. If a client does not trust you and you try to pry details of painful, life-altering incidents from them, it is unlikely that you will ever develop a productive – and helpful – therapeutic relationship.*

When Beef was nine, he committed some act, a small, childish prank, which led to more than the usual beating. His mother had him removed again, this time to some sort of home for boys. I never saw Beef cry, but whenever he talked about this, his whole countenance sagged. He momentarily lost his poise, the matter-of-fact swagger he used to describe the most terrible moments of his life. He told me how he cried and begged his mother not to send him away and how frightened he was. "I was just a little kid…and I was a good kid up to that time. She took that away from me."

"A good kid..." that is how Beef saw himself. I once asked him to describe himself to me. He said he was a good person, adding, "I care about others." He did not see the dangerous killer others saw.

Beef never said much about the Boys home. A characteristic of trauma victims is that they depersonalize a lot, often fantasizing to avoid the pain. Beef always changed the topic, only rarely allowing me to enter that painful part of his past. He could be very good at disclosing small, private and sometimes even embarrassing details of his life, especially his crimes, but the painful things were often forgotten, pushed from his thoughts to a secret place where no one else could go. One telling incident did come to light, though. During a work detail at the Boys school, Beef assaulted one of the staff. He was punished by being forced to lie in a field, tied down on his back for hours in the hot sun. He claimed to have suffered permanent eye damage from this. He always wore sunglasses and stated that this was the reason. He was ten or eleven years old when this occurred.

When Beef was released at age twelve, he returned to his mother and the man he calls his father. He does not know if this man is indeed his father, but he does remember the beatings. One day, a few months after his return, his father was drunk and beating his mother and sister. Beef took his father's revolver and shot him through the stomach. He did not die but Beef got sent back to an institution once again. He later told me, in a rather matter-of-fact manner, that he and his father are still in contact. "I crippled him...but he knows he deserved it. He didn't beat anyone else." Beef was released at age thirteen and returned to his mother's custody. It was around this time that he and his mother, along with his sister and baby brother, moved to Massachusetts. By now, Beef's life was enmeshed with his mother's life – one of drug use, abusive relationships and apparent mental illness. But he worshipped his little sister and appears to have made it his job to protect her.

Beef described his mother as, "always working," but he never used that phrase to mean employment. He used "work" to describe her way of using people - boyfriends, strangers, landlords, neighbors and her own children. He related an incident in which he "skipped out" of a work release program prior to completion of his second life sentence. He moved into an abandoned house next to his mother's and "holed up" with a bottle of whiskey and some drugs. His mother gave him a gun, telling him it was for his own protection. Then she called the police and told them that he was armed and wanted to shoot it out with them. A SWAT team surrounded the house and Beef was forced to strip naked and come out with his hands in the air or the police would kill him. "The bitch had insurance on me and she wanted to collect...she's always working."

Beef related another incident, at the time he was just a child, when his mother owned a rooming house and would rent to transients and other poor. One day, one of her tenants died in his room. "My mother made me go in and empty out the old man's pockets and take his wallet and money. I hated touching that dead old man. He smelled. I hate dead bodies to this day. The bitch made me do it." Mom was working again.

As Beef entered his adolescent years, he became increasingly angry. His self-image was terrible and he viewed the world only as a hostile place. His mother, when she was not drinking or doing drugs, was busy working some scheme for money, rarely giving anything but negative attention to her brood. Children are not miniature adults and when hurt they will act out by transferring their pain and rejection onto others. Beef was always told he was bad, so before long he saw himself that way and his mother's words became self-fulfilling. At age fourteen, Beef started to vent his anger on strangers. He told me how he used to stab winos, the old drunks and homeless that populated his neighborhood. He explained his actions like this, "Whenever it started to build up...my anger...I'd go find some wino. It didn't matter if they were awake or passed out. I just felt better when I cut them. I didn't kill none of them...they're only winos. Nobody gives a shit about them anyway."

Just before he turned 15, Beef's mother shipped him to a relative in Alabama. There, shortly after his 15th birthday, he stabbed a man to death in a drug deal gone bad. Tried as an adult, he was sentenced to life in prison.

Beef's life made him a survivor. Smart, young, tough and quickly wise to prison life, he learned to present an attitude that sent a message – and that was, "Don't screw with me or I'll kill you." He joined a prison gang and learned how to use people but was badly used himself. Much of his time served was "bad" time. He was placed in solitary confinement for months on end and was kept in maximum security for much of his prison time. After fifteen years, he was paroled. "They gave me a ticket back to Massachusetts and told me never to return." Beef was now thirty years old and back with his mother. His little brother was serving time in New York for rape. His sister was living somewhere in Florida. Beef joked, "At least we traveled." Beef had spent all his adult life and most of his youth in some type of institution. He was not exactly dressed for success. But he met a woman and, within a year of his release had fathered a daughter.

If Beef had a chance, it was during this period. He lived with a girlfriend and, through a state sponsored program, was learning to work with troubled youth. In spite of his history, Beef was intelligent and motivated to do something right. However, old habits are hard to break – and drug habits can be unbreakable. Shortly after his daughter was born, Beef found heroin. It was to be expected. He came from a world of gangs, drugs and violence and returned from prison less equipped to handle life than when he entered. His drug habit got worse and soon his girlfriend left him and took the baby. He moved back with his mother who encouraged him to steal. When Beef described this to me, he went to great pains to explain that his mother logically figured that since he was going to steal to support his drug habit, better to steal from others than from her. Anyway, Mom got first dibs on his stolen goods and would help him fence the rest.

Beef was also becoming increasingly psychotic. His past abuse, the abandonment, the losses, the isolation, and the lack of living skills coupled with a growing heroin addiction turned Beef into a time bomb. On a Summer night in the early 1970's, the time bomb detonated. Beef went to a convenience store to collect a drug debt. The store had money and two people behind the counter. Beef shot them both. He did not just march in shooting, however. He made them close the store, took them into the back room where he forced them to kneel and say their prayers and shot both men in the head.

Beef was sentenced to two consecutive life terms in a Maximum-Security State Prison. This effectively eliminated any chance of Beef ever again being free. During the trial, a reporter interviewed his mother. She played the victim card well. She told the reporter that Reynold was always a problem and she did not know why God had given her such a burden. She was working again.

It was in State Prison that Reynold became known as "Beef." His sense of pride was obvious when he talked about his time there. "They never broke me...they couldn't break me like they broke others. They broke my brother, drove him nuts...he was crying and babbling like a baby."

It was here that Beef honed his skills, learning to fight and to kill. He claimed that he killed five other inmates during his time there. He spent a lot of time in "the hole," in solitary confinement. He claims, although I have no way to verify any of this, that he spent more consecutive time in the hole than any man ever did in Maximum Security–over five straight years. He explained that he had taken part in a prison strike. He and the other leaders of it were locked in solitary confinement until they admitted their roles in the uprising. "One guy lasted 18 months before breaking down." Beef claims he never budged. I am unsure if his description of "the hole" is accurate, but other clients who had been there verified much of his description. "The hole" is described as an empty cell with a metal bench and a hole in the floor to use as a toilet. "They have to provide you with a mattress, but they come and take it away from you about 3:00 AM." Food is slipped to you through a hole in the door, and Beef always claimed the "screws" (guards) spit in it. There is no TV, no radio and no windows, only a solitary light that is left on for 24 hours. He once told me, "I could sometimes tell when it was raining or snowing by the way the screws were dressed." Beef also said that there was a camera watching you constantly. He laughed as he told me how he would face the camera and masturbate, his own way of telling the screws what he thought of them. For exercise, the inmates got to walk outside in a small enclosure twice a week, followed by a twice-weekly shower.

Once, during one of our meetings, I asked Beef how he kept from losing his mind after being there for so long. He told me that a prison social worker taught him how to meditate and described it in detail, adding that it kept him from going crazy. He said, "Each morning after they fed me, I would get comfortable sitting on the floor. I would start by staring at the wall and counting the rivets around the door. I would stare at them until they all kind of went blank, and it got quiet. Then, I could go anywhere I wanted. I'd first go to a stream in the woods...lots of trees and water. I remember seeing a place like that once when I was a kid. It got easy to do...it was my way to get out. I escaped that way in my head. That's why they couldn't break me. Each day I escaped. When they brought my lunch, I'd snap out of it. Sometime they'd have to yell at me, like they thought something was wrong. But I wasn't there. After I ate, I'd shit and then start yelling and raising hell like everyone else. I'd already been outside."

Beef served 18 years of his double life sentence. Acting as his own lawyer for much of his appeal process, his double life was commuted to a single, second-degree conviction, making him eligible for parole. Out less than a year and outside of an institution for less than three years in the past 35, Beef was on methadone to overcome his heroin dependence and was smoking crack cocaine daily when we met. Oh yes, he was again living with his mother. Working with Beef provided one of my greatest challenges.

Beef did not have a lot of trouble kicking heroin. He had not been using steadily for too long, so he reached a *therapeutic methadone dosage, (def.) one at which he felt neither withdrawal nor the need for more heroin* and was starting to enjoy being free. He liked being outside in good weather but otherwise spent much of his day, "doing his bit" at home, under the watchful eye of his mother. I was initially unaware of his mother's role in his addiction and mental health issues, but I soon found out.

Beef liked to take long walks alone at night. When he first told me this, I asked if he did not think walking around the streets of Worcester at night was kind of dangerous, after all, his neighborhood was not exactly the place one wants to find himself stranded alone. What could I have been thinking? Beef gave a rare grin and said, "I'm a lot more dangerous than anyone else out there." A few years later, I saw the Disney movie, "Shrek" about an ogre, a monster of fairy tales. In the movie, the ogre makes much the same comment about walking through woods filled with thieves and wolves, saying, "I'm scarier than anything else out there." He should have met Beef.

Beef got a little aggravated when the local police would stop him almost nightly to check his ID and ask what he was doing out. He figured it was a racial thing. Actually, anyone White, Black or otherwise was likely to be stopped by police in that neighborhood walking alone at night. Once, Beef described a lone police officer pulling up beside him in a cruiser. The police officer remained in his vehicle and asked Beef for his ID. "He didn't even bother to get out…he was real careless. If I was high, I could have killed him and kept walking. No one would have even known."

Shortly before entering the methadone program, Beef renewed an old prison contact who introduced him to crack cocaine, which was cheap and easy to get. Crack use is as close to instant addiction as you can find. (We will look at cocaine in more detail later.) Beef realized however, that his continued use of cocaine would eventually get him sent back to prison, so he wanted to quit. It was in this way that I learned about his mother. Mom was "always working" to make sure he stayed under her control. She used his cocaine habit to keep it that way.

Crack cocaine (def.) is small pieces of cocaine hydrochloride base that have been chemically separated from its impurities. When processed, it becomes brittle and is cracked into pieces which are heated and smoked. Hence, the name "crack." It is usually sold in "rocks," the small pieces of cocaine base. At this time a rock was selling for about $20.00. Beef's mother would make sure that he had exactly $20.00 every morning when he left the house. Even when he wanted to quit, she gave him the money and told him, "…it's okay, just so long as you come straight home to smoke it."

Chronic cocaine use causes psychosis in many individuals. Beef was already carrying a history of this diagnosis and a scary track record to prove it. It was Martin Luther King Day when his controls came loose.

MLK Day is a federal holiday celebrated on Monday, but methadone clinics do not close on this or any other day. My wife had a doctor's appointment later that week so I decided that I would work the Monday holiday and take a day off later to be with her. Other than the nurses who were locked in the dispensing area handing out methadone, I was the only other person in the building. Beef had been using crack cocaine daily and we had been working together on behavior modification techniques to help him kick it. That Monday morning, however, Beef looked and sounded different.

One of the skills you develop working with addicts is kind of a sixth sense that helps you recognize quickly when something is not right. It is like another learned skill that enables you to know when a client is afraid of discussing something or is avoiding telling you about a painful event from his past. I once heard it called *hearing the unspoken word*. It is somewhat instinctual, requiring you to pick up non-verbal cues and innuendoes quickly.

Beef, like a lot of ex-convicts, always made poor eye contact. Perhaps looking someone in the eye is viewed as aggression. Honestly, I never really gave it a lot of thought. Beef always had his sunglasses on anyway, so I was used to not making good eye contact with him. This day, however, he was not wearing his glasses and was watching me closely. And the first words out of him hinted at hostility. "Why are you working on Brother Martin's Day?" Normally, I would have made an excuse, explaining it away quickly and getting on with whatever topic was at hand. My sixth sense kicked in however and I was immediately cautious. Actually, I told Beef the truth.

During this period, my wife was terminally ill. Some of my clients were aware of this since I sometimes needed to take time off with sudden cancellations or rescheduled appointments. In addition, I had been called out of work for emergencies multiple times and word got out quickly that my wife was sick. I explained the situation to Beef, adding that I would take MLK Day off later in the week. That answer satisfied him. He told me he could not stand anyone disrespecting Reverend King. He then went on to tell me he was "really pissed off" and that bad feelings had been building all week. He detailed how he no longer cared about anything, not even if the police killed him. He had a girlfriend in a nearby town who had a gun for him and he was going to go get it. Pursuing this further, I asked him what he intended to do. "I need to kill someone." His emphasis was on "need."

Beef then described much of the same build-up of anger and paranoia that he had related to me weeks earlier when telling me about stabbing winos. We spent a long time together that day, far longer than the usual 50-minute session, about two hours. Beef talked about how, in prison, he always had a "shiv," a homemade knife, and how he used to force others to do his bidding. He spoke quite graphically about beating, raping and abusing other inmates, "dogs," when things began to build up inside him, as was happening at this time.

Looking back on this now, I realize I was "winging it," but I knew I had to keep Beef talking and engaged with me until I figured out what I had to do to get him under control again. I pointed out to Beef that his thinking was different this day and he sounded depressed. I put a label – depression – on what was bothering him, and he listened. I also pointed out to him that he sounded very suspicious of everyone around him. And I told him I was worried about him. (He would later tell me that he appreciated hearing that most of all.) I told him that he needed to stop using cocaine *now*, not tomorrow or some other time, but now. I also told him that I would get him some medication to help him.

Holidays are not the easiest time to get hold of a psychiatrist, but I got lucky. The only one Beef would agree to see was Dr. A., our clinic psychiatrist. On a chance, I called Worcester's St. Vincent Hospital and found Dr. A. making rounds. He agreed to see Beef at once. In a few minutes, Beef was on his way to the hospital.

I am grateful that this day worked out the way it did. Beef later told me that he intended to kill someone and probably would have. It could have been me or, more likely, it would have been an innocent person who crossed his path. *I have always maintained that no therapist can take the blame when a client relapses and destroys something because we cannot take the credit when one succeeds.* However, I likely would have blamed myself if I could not have stopped him that day and he murdered someone. After Beef left, I quite literally said a prayer of thanks.

Within a few weeks, Beef was free from cocaine and was being maintained on anti-psychotic medications. I continued to see him for another two years, working through a difficult reunification with his daughter, who was by now a local college student, and through the accidental overdose death of a girlfriend. Through none of this did Beef suffer either a drug relapse or another psychotic episode. Oh yes, he moved out of his mother's house too.

***

There are times when I find myself getting a little philosophical as to what makes the difference in the lives of people living in a world of abuse, neglect and drugs. Why can some recover while others cannot make it despite great effort and expense? Some, like

Manny, recover despite overwhelming odds. Others, like Beef, survive and eventually recover but leave wrecked lives in their wake. Some will repeat the mistakes of their parents and others will pass through life exhibiting a litany of mental health disorders. Still others seem to function better, becoming over-achievers and successful. What is undeniable is that those born into a world of addiction, as well as those who stumble into it through bad companions, immaturity or naivete' will be scarred physically, socially and mentally and their values will be trashed – and those who recover will do so only by making **change.** Tragically, not all are able to make the necessary changes and some do not even recognize there is a problem. Later, we will look closely at what constitutes *the changes necessary to overcome addiction.*

Finally, it should also be noted here that Beef was diagnosed as suffering from a Personality Disorder, (*def.*): *a long-term pattern of thoughts and behaviors that differ from what is considered normal and occurs since age 15 years.* Specifically, with his lengthy history of criminal and violent behavior, Beef was described as a sociopath, and as such, met the diagnostic criteria for an Antisocial Personality Disorder (301.7). Those diagnosed with this disorder are described as lacking insight into their behavior and having no conscience. However, clean and free of illicit drugs, Beef's anti-social traits diminished and he was able to develop both insight into his behavior and the ability to live and function in his world. As I complete this book, fifteen years have passed and Beef remains clean and sober.

Summary:

Addiction is generational, with most addicts having at least one addicted parent. There are many factors influencing the development of an addiction, including but not limited to, learned, environmental, behavioral and genetic influences. Chief among these are negative parental factors such as unhealthy example, abuse, neglect and trauma. Also prominent are mental health issues such as depression, anxiety and personality disorders.

For those involved with treating an addict, whether as a therapist or a medical professional, the building of trust is the primary concern for developing a relationship. Most addicts have histories of neglect or trauma, some far worse than others. Many addicts carry unresolved guilt issues due to their actions. Many others have behaviors that can be violent or controlled, manipulative or submissive. Addicts with a history of trauma have difficulty with relationships, love, trust and communication. They frequently depersonalize and fantasize to escape their traumatic memories. These behaviors are survival techniques learned by the addict early in life and can make addressing trauma extremely difficult, since the addict's inability to trust is compounded by the drive to escape painful memories.

*Those who recover from addictions do so by making **behavioral changes – for example, changes in how they cope, respond to stress, socialize and set personal goals.** These changes often begin when an honest, trusting relationship between therapist and addict develops.*

Many addicts suffering from personality disorders find that they become less dominant as recovery from addiction continues.

CHAPTER 2:
GETTING TO KNOW YOU

I began my career in addiction treatment in the early1970's as an entry-level counselor in a Worcester, Massachusetts alcoholism treatment program called Doctors Hospital, today called AdCare. It combined a detoxification unit and inpatient counseling program with follow up psychotherapy and social services. *Detoxification, or "detox" (def.) is the medical process of removing the physiological effects of either alcohol and/or drugs which have been smoked, snorted, injected, eaten, inhaled or otherwise ingested from a patient's system while minimizing serious withdrawal and side effects.*

For most, a detox is no big deal. A few tranquilizers, some sleep and a little good food and the patient is often ready to go out and do it all over again. Unfortunately, many did just that. At Doctors Hospital, the staff and the chronic repeaters were on a first name basis. One of them, very typical of an inner-city population, was Henry, your stereotypical, skid-row bum, emaciated, scarred and brain damaged. Once a well-paid steel worker, homeowner and father of a grown family, Henry landed on skid row after the demise of the local steel plant. Plant closings put Henry and many like him on the skids. *Working with Henry made me realize how closely skid row lies for many of us.*

Henry proudly stated, "I never missed a day of work in 20 years." I have no way of knowing whether this was true, but Henry worked at the local steel mill for over 25 years with an excellent record. But Henry never saw it coming – and I do not just mean the plant closing.

Like most of his friends and co-workers, Henry went to a neighborhood club after work each afternoon. There, he drank a few beers and went home. After the plant shut down, Henry got to the club earlier and earlier each day. Soon, instead of getting there after work, he arrived in the morning. The club became the support system where he met his friends, talked about his troubles and cultivated his growing dependence on alcohol. Not only did Henry never see it coming, he never even knew when it ran right over him. After all, how could he have a problem with his drinking? He never missed work, he had a family, he paid his bills and he did not drink any more than everyone else he knew.

One day Millie, his wife of 30 years, tossed him out. Too much booze, too nasty too often, drinking up the money and now the kids were becoming ashamed of their father. It built up gradually. To Henry, it came without warning. Henry found his bags packed and the police at the door. Millie did not give him a choice.

Where does a man go at a time like that? His siblings had their own families and could not handle or did not want Henry, so he did the most natural thing. He got a room in a downtown Worcester rooming house, close to his friends at the club. There was no turning back.

I was picking my mother up from a local hospital after surgery a few years ago. She was being discharged a day early so she could be home for Thanksgiving. As I was getting ready to sign Mom out, I looked up and spied Henry walking out of a room across the hall. It had been a couple of years, but he remembered me. Of course, he also knew I was an easy mark for a little pocket change. Anyway, after chatting a few minutes, I asked a nurse how Henry was doing. She looked so sympathetic telling me, "Such a nice old gentleman...but he fell out of bed last night and hurt his hip. He's probably stuck here through the holiday." I did not have the heart to tell her that Henry fell out of bed in every hospital in Worcester County. It was usually just before discharge and right before the holidays. That hip had been bad for years. (Henry was also hit by a bus and a taxi and God only knows what else. That hip earned more money than he did.) For Henry, like many others, being in a hospital or a detox over the holidays beat having to go back to a lonely room watching reruns with a bottle of wine.

One of the young physicians who rotated through Doctors Hospital wrote a lengthy and rather compassionate note in Henry's medical record. He described how Henry had only been exhibiting signs of alcoholism for "a few years" (actually, by this time it had been well over a decade.) He suggested that Henry should be kept inpatient a little longer so that someone in social services could contact his wife and try to arrange a family reunification. The poor doctor was offended when everyone laughed at him. Henry called Millie regularly and we would hear him giving her "one more chance" to take him back. The staff, myself included, became cynical dealing with people like Henry who just never improved. We laughed at his attempts to control a life that had spun irrevocably out of control. Someone once said that if you do not laugh, you will cry. Perhaps. But laughter at another person's pain is cruelty. And we all knew better. I am truly sorry for seeing humor in Henry's suffering. Henry never got visits from Millie nor from his three children. No cards, no calls, no visits. He died alone.

Henry was found dead in a doorway not far from the Public Inebriate Program, the PIP Shelter, as it was known. His pockets were empty and there was a nasty bump on his head. No one even bothered to consider that he might have died as a result of being mugged. It was almost a week before anyone identified his body.

***

Admissions to detox always increase around the holidays. Street people, elderly addicts and others who have burned their bridges find the holidays to be tough. Toss down a bottle of wine, show up at detox and you wake up in a warm room with clean sheets and good food. There was a strange, family-like atmosphere as patients gathered in the hospital's kitchenette drinking coffee, swapping stories and drying out. Christmas morning in detox might be lonely, but it beat being alone.

The holidays are tough for those new in recovery, but can bring out small acts of nobility. Many can be found manning the kitchen at free charity dinners that crop up to serve the "less fortunate." Even those with little to give and less to be thankful for find that sharing what they have provides something they have been unsuccessfully seeking through chemicals – it makes them feel good.

Juanita was a long-time heroin addict with a track record of dope dealing, jail time and homelessness. Born in Spanish Harlem, an addict at 15, prostitution at the hands of a "boyfriend" at 16 and her three children lost to Child Protective Services, she had little to be thankful for. Somewhere along the way though, Juanita met and married a man who treated her right and hung in there through her periodic drug binges. I met Juanita in the mid 1980's early in her recovery. It was just before Christmas that year when her husband, "Johnny" bought her a lottery ticket and Juanita won $1,000.00. Now, when an addict comes into easy money, even a modest sum like this, it is usually a ticket to the next binge. Not this time though. Juanita went to a local church where she found a "giving tree" filled with the names of children from needy families along with a request for a toy or an article of clothing. Juanita took all the names from the tree and spent every cent on gifts for the children. When I asked her about this, her eyes glistened and she pointed to her heart, saying in her broken English, "It made me feel good right here." I must admit, it made me feel good that day too.

My first patient as *Counselor 1* was Mr. George Coleman. He was in the detoxification unit, having just arrived the previous night. Being a novice to the business, I was more than a little nervous about meeting my first patient. He was lying on his bed with his eyes closed so I gently touched his foot and inquired, "Mr. Coleman?" He instantly woke up, sat up and threw up – although not completely in that order. It is called projectile vomiting. He hit the sheets, the floor and the wall beyond the foot of his bed, which I figure was about an eight-foot shot. "Jesus Christ George, you hit everything but Broadway," one of the nurses growled. I shall always be thankful that I was standing beside his bed and not at the foot of it. Somehow, perhaps it was Mr. Coleman's total lack of concern about his puking, or anything else for that matter, or maybe it was the "who gives a shit" attitude in response to little crises like this, but I was never nervous again. I drove home that day thinking, "I'm gonna like this job."

George never mentioned the incident, he probably could not remember it anyway, but during one of his later stays in detox, he told me that when he first met me, he thought to himself, "Who is this asshole?" Now though, he did not think I was an asshole. So much for compliments.

***

Death is a regular occurrence when working with addictions. It leaves you feeling powerless when you are sitting with someone, often a very young and very bright person, whom you know is going to die because he or she cannot stop getting high. You want so badly to say the right words that, like magic, will make that person want to get clean and sober. This desire often served to make me overly optimistic about everyone's chances, believing that even the most hopeless case could get clean if I said the right words. I still find it hard to accept the fact that some people just have to die from their addictions.

AGAINST ALL ODDS

Treatment is certainly not all death and dying. One of the most important realizations about recovery is that nothing builds character like getting knocked down repeatedly by drugs or alcohol. It forces personal growth and an often much-needed self-examination. It confirms my observation that some of those I worked with were among the finest people I have ever met.

For his 50th birthday, Wes Black was, "...in that f**kin' loony bin," as he affectionately called a local psychiatric unit. He was broke, homeless and minus his second wife. His kids wanted nothing to do with him and he was not only unemployed but had been blackballed from his career. Wes had lost it all. Within a few weeks he went from being a highly successful corporate executive with a million-dollar home and all the toys to homelessness. I spent a lot of time with Wes as he grieved his losses while trying to make amends and crawl back from the pit he found himself in. On his final binge, Wes tried to take his own life by driving his car into a lake. He got stuck in the mud and was arrested for driving under the influence, after which he was committed to a local psychiatric unit for his own protection. When arrested, he told the police he wanted to die and said, "See, I can't even do that right."

After getting out of the psychiatric ward, Wes went to court to answer for his misdeeds. The judge chuckled and said he should have been arrested for polluting the pond instead. He was then let off with probation and a suspended sentence. There are times when a break like that can make a difference. This was one of them. Wes promised the judge he would do his best and he indeed kept his promise. Wes never drank or used illicit drugs again.

Wes's emotional pain was almost palpable. He loved his wife and felt abandoned by her at a time when he was finally putting his life back together. However, it is a terrible realization for a man, or a woman for that matter, that they are better off without their biggest excuse for relapsing. Wes likely would have relapsed had he returned to his wife. She was a lot younger and he had met her in a bar. It was not a healthy situation to begin with, and it took a couple of years for him to realize it. Wes worked through the anger, the tears and the loneliness. He went through alcohol and cannabis withdrawal and then the post-acute withdrawal syndrome. *Post-acute withdrawal syndrome (def.) is a condition experienced by many who quit alcohol and/or drug use. It leaves its victims depressed, moody and suffering from insomnia, sometime for months after they have stopped using. It manifests primarily as emotional issues, mood swings and impaired decision making.* But for Wes, the process worked, for somewhere he heard what he needed to hear in order to change his behaviors.

Early in his recovery, an old timer in a self-help group told Wes, "Any asshole can stop drinking but *you* are going to get sober." He did not quite know what this meant but he stopped drinking and smoking marijuana. He went to all kinds of support meetings. He listened and learned – and he changed. This is what terms like "getting sober" and "recovery" are all about. *It is not just putting aside drugs and alcohol, it is growing up, changing, evolving into something better. It is important to understand that those who successfully recover from addictions make significant changes to their lifestyle beyond simply quitting their chemical use.*

"I hang in there in spite of the bastards," Wes was fond of saying. "The bastards" were those who predicted failure, who laughed at the changes he made, and those whose trust of Wes had long since disappeared. Some of his old business associates refused to talk to him, sending the message that he was beyond recovery. He spent his first holidays alone, attending an "Alcathon" a 24-hour Alcoholics Anonymous meeting held over Christmas that year. His family did not want him around to spoil their holiday. Gradually however, Wes made amends to his family and began to hold his head up despite their rejection.

Today, Wes has a new business and employs his youngest son. He is pushing seventy years old but still works twelve-hour days. He spends time with his grandchildren and even finds time for a little romance, so he tells me. He is happy. He changed, becoming more than just some "asshole who'd quit drinking." He got sober. A few years ago, Wes quoted one of the clichés he heard at a support group meeting. He said it sums up his recovery. "I ain't what I would be; I ain't what I should be; I ain't what I could be. But at least I ain't what I used to be."

TO HELL AND BACK

The chances of Luis Monfreda achieving recovery were next to zero. The middle child of five, he was born in a Brooklyn tenement to a Hispanic family where drinking and fighting were the norm. His parents split when he was about nine years old. He remained with his mother, who moved her brood to what was arguably the most dangerous section of New York, the South Bronx. Throughout the 1970's, the South Bronx was the urban renewal poster child. A cavernous neighborhood of noise and grime, it became the backdrop for every local and national politician who wanted to point out the failures of the prior administration. It was also the setting for many Hollywood productions depicting violent city gangs, squalid neighborhoods, racial warfare and crooked cops. The South Bronx failed to improve through a lot of political administrations, while much of the neighborhood acquired the look of bombed-out Berlin at the end of World War II.

Luis played in the run-down streets, abandoned buildings and lots filled with stripped cars. In the summer, the city broiled as the blacktop, bricks and tarred roofs absorbed the sun. Luis described how his mother would put the children in a bathtub full of cold water in front of a fan. He called it "ghetto air conditioning." Come the fall, the wind would howl through the vacant buildings and the streets became bitter. Luis hated how his nose would run and his lips and cheeks became raw and red. "They felt like someone sandpapered them." Schools in the Bronx reflected poverty with never enough books, nor enough teachers for that matter. He attended school when he felt like it and, like many, he could barely read. His combined English/Spanish environment did nothing to foster his reading skills nor to understand or care about the world around him. Luis had no positive role models and the only successes he saw were pimps and drug dealers driving their big cars.

Then Luis found something that made him feel accepted and cared for more than his family. At age 12, Luis joined a gang. Like his two older brothers, he learned to guard his turf. He learned to fight and to steal. And he learned to use drugs. Everybody used marijuana. He said that, at one time in his life, he knew no one who did not at least smoke pot. There were other drugs too, heroin, cocaine, amphetamines and assorted pills. He even tried methadone, although he did not see what the big deal was. All this by the time he was 15 years old.

By the time Luis reached mid-adolescence, he was an accomplished car thief. Small, wiry and fast, he kept one step ahead of the law, somehow avoiding reform school (or any other school for that matter.) It was during this time however, that Luis was most dangerous. Eager to prove himself as a gang member, he carried a knife and began mugging those who would be foolish enough to leave themselves vulnerable in those dark, inner-city streets. This included lost strangers, drunks or junkies too stoned to fight back as well as members of other gangs who strayed into the wrong part of the city. Luis got his first life-threatening wound on one of these late-night forays. Knifed in the liver and lungs, he nearly bled to death. After that incident, his mother sent him to live with his father.

Luis's father and mother had split up after his father came home drunk one night and beat his wife bloody for some long-forgotten offense. He stopped drinking soon afterwards when he "found Jesus" in a Salvation Army shelter. The following four years were good to Luis's father. He quit drinking, opened a store-front diner, worked hard and expanded it into a moderately successful Spanish-American restaurant. The neighborhood was better, still inner city, but with fewer transients and gangs. It was to his father's home that Luis now moved.

One thing had not changed. His father still ruled with a heavy hand. He had another wife by now and resented taking Luis into his home – and Luis felt that resentment daily. As time went on however, Luis bonded with his father's new wife, for both were frequent targets of the man's anger. Many years later, Luis would recognize that for him, recovery meant, "…using my mind and my heart, not my fists…My father dried out without ever really changing. I had to do better than that." In many conversations about his dad, Luis grew to understand his father and more importantly, to forgive him.

At age 16, Luis fathered his first child, Little Luis. Luis talked often of his children. He fathered four by three different women. The values of my Caucasian middle-class upbringing tend to judge this quite harshly. Perhaps it is necessary to grow up in a ghetto, be nurtured by a gang and know nothing beyond the blacktopped despair of violence and addiction to understand the need to create and love something that needs and loves you back.

Luis always kept in touch with his oldest son and expressed a lot of anguish when, as a teenager, the boy moved to Puerto Rico with his mother. Luis reached out however, and Little Luis responded. They still call each other weekly.

The move to his father's house only put a temporary halt to Luis's slide. He continued with gang involvement and the gang became more violent. The 1970's brought on a new and increased volatility to inner cities with an economic recession, increased drug use and public officials at a loss over how to address the situation. Luis knew nothing of the world or of society around him. He only knew that he needed to make money to feed a growing drug dependence. As an adolescent, Luis first experimented with, and then regularly used heroin. Intravenous drug use was a part of his world. By 1980, now a young man with a habit, Luis graduated to bigger things. He started carrying a gun and became an armed robber.

It was a blessing of sorts that Luis was not a good armed robber. He did mostly "smash and grab" jobs, crashing a display case to steal the cigarettes or grabbing a handful of bills from an open cash register. When he tried moving up to robbing a liquor store, a police officer was waiting and shot him. After a few weeks in the hospital, Luis got five years in prison.

There is nothing pleasant about incarceration. Luis spoke little of the experience, something I found common to most who have done time. Maybe it is the brutality or maybe it is the boredom of being in a cell day after day. Perhaps some are just ashamed of having been there. Luis, like most, just never brought it up. One good thing occurred in prison however. Luis got an education. As part of his rehabilitation, Luis learned to study and got his high school diploma. Just as important, Luis learned that there is a world that existed outside of the city. Shortly after his parole in 1983, Luis met his first wife. Gloria was tall and beautiful. She was also smart, insisting that they move away from the city. They moved to a rural setting in Western Massachusetts where Luis got a factory job and they began to build a life together.

It is said that children are a blank slate upon which their life experiences are printed. Luis's slate was stamped from infancy with violence and drug use. As a result, Luis found himself ill-equipped to handle the pressures of life in the suburbs. He had no close friends, no support system and no healthy ways to vent frustrations, fears and problems. He became short-tempered and irritable. His drinking had become excessive by the time Gloria gave birth to their second child, another boy. The drinking escalated and one day Luis struck Gloria with his fist.

Domestic violence is arguably the most generational of society's problems. Luis learned it as a child from his father, who in turn had learned it from his. Later, Luis would tell me, "I became my father…a workaholic with a beer and an ugly temper."

Gloria stayed for a while. She heard his apologies, the "I'm sorry…I don't know why I did it…I just lost it…It won't happen again…I love you." Words that became increasingly empty. Luis even stopped drinking for a while. After a Superbowl party one cold February night however, Luis and Gloria argued. He again drank and he again struck her.

Marriages, like all relationships, are built upon three legs. The first is love, including both the physical and emotional contact, the second is trust and the third is respect. Domestic violence pretty much wipes out all three. How does a woman trust and respect the person who abuses her? How does someone stay with an explosive spouse, always "waiting for the other shoe to drop?" Where is respect when a person uses violence and intimidation to coerce and control the one they claim to love? What domestic violence does not kill, alcohol and drug abuse will finish off. Gloria packed up and left, taking their two sons, now toddlers, with her.

It was now that the cruelest irony struck. Gloria moved in with a man who used cocaine intravenously. Gloria had never used anything beyond marijuana. This man introduced her to cocaine,

45

then to a needle to administer it. The year was 1984. At that time, a terrifying illness was making headlines daily - AIDS.

Luis got clean and sober once again and joined a support group. After a few months, Gloria returned to him and attended meetings with him. The damage was done however. Over the next few years Gloria got sick, increasingly weak and died of AIDS just before Christmas in 1990. Luis remained at her side, sober and attentive. He nursed Gloria and became a gentle, loyal husband, in love with her until the end. But the penance for his own past sins was also Acquired Immune Deficiency Syndrome, now called Human Immunodeficiency Virus or HIV, named more appropriately for the virus, not just the symptoms.

After Gloria's death, Luis suspected that he too had contracted HIV. He woke with night sweats and nausea and was losing weight. Facing this and alone with his grief when Gloria's family took custody of his two boys, Luis did what an addict does. He got high. He told me later through tears that he never felt so totally alone. Luis stayed high to avoid the pain. He committed petty crimes and dealt dope to other addicts to support his habit. After two lost months, Luis landed in front of a judge who sent him into treatment. It was while detoxing in 1991 that he met a girl named Maritza.

As a detoxification is completed, most people start to feel well again and find that their emotions and hormones have returned with a vengeance. So, the first person who smiles at them is often the first person they fall in love with. This is almost never good news, for detox romances rarely survive the first crisis.

Maritza is a pretty, hot-tempered girl from Puerto Rico. She was homeless with a three-year old son, a diagnosis of HIV and a heroin addiction. She was close to losing her son to foster care and had no idea where, how, or even if she could ever find a stable way to live. Then Maritza met Luis, who always seemed to have the odds stacked against him. The chance of this relationship lasting beyond the first relapse was zero. Their combined drug habits, HIV diagnoses and backgrounds of abuse virtually eliminated any chance of success. So, of course, Luis and Maritza have somehow beaten the odds and made it work.

In their first month together, Luis confirmed his suspicions and received his diagnosis of HIV. Immediately, as was to be expected upon hearing the news, he relapsed, taking Maritza on a binge with him. They found themselves homeless again and living in a succession of shelters while the state put her son back into foster care with one of Maritza's aunts. Maritza then became pregnant. Somehow, at a time when things could not have gotten worse, this marked the point when this unlikely couple began to turn things around.

Maritza remained healthy, took AZT (*def.*) *Azidothymidine, the first successful anti-viral medication for HIV treatment, also called Zidovudine and Retrovir*) and the little girl that arrived tested negative for "the virus," as HIV was commonly called. (This was prior to the Covid 19 virus, a pandemic that has now usurped the label, *the virus.*) Luis also began taking anti-viral meds and, more importantly, began his recovery in earnest. He started receiving a disability check and Maritza got a job. Between them, this provided enough to get an apartment and Maritza eventually got her son back. Both entered long-term methadone treatment. It was here that I began working with Luis while Maritza worked with one of my colleagues in counseling at the methadone clinic. He and Maritza were already clean almost six months and were on *methadone maintenance,* a form of treatment what can conceivably last a lifetime. *Methadone maintenance (def.) provides long-term therapeutic dosing with methadone that keeps withdrawal symptoms away while blocking the effects of other opioids like heroin. The dosage remains stable, is low cost, is covered by many third-party payers and is effective for many long-term addicts. Methadone is usually dispensed daily at clinics, requiring in-person visits, random blood tests and regular, usually weekly, counseling.* Luis weaned off methadone over a three-year period, all while working to improve and strengthen his recovery.

Luis began to immediately work at accepting his diseases – both of them – HIV and addiction. He occasionally quoted something he heard at a support group, and it was one of the first things he told me, "I will not live one second longer than God intends me to." He was actually quoting the late Egyptian President Anwar Sadat, but added, "God put me here for a reason, so I need to live as long as I can." Luis fully understood that if he wanted to live, he needed to learn about his diseases and what needed to be done physically and mentally to stay healthy. Today, he takes his medications, exercises, rests and meditates. He also quit smoking and watches his diet.

Another recovery tool, meditation, helps Luis handle his emotional stressors and problems effectively. He uses meditation in much the same way others use religion. *Meditation (def.) helps a person eliminate unnecessary stimuli from their mind, so that focus can be more centered.* Meditation has helped Luis to focus on relaxation and strengthen his recovery. It let Luis clarify his beliefs and build his own spirituality. Luis did not have a whole lot of formal religion – he still does not. But what he has is spirituality, a trait found in many of those with successful recovery. Luis once told me, "Religion is what you find in people who are afraid of going to Hell. Spirituality is what you find in people who've already been there." I thought that was pretty good insight.

Luis is not a churchgoer, does not thump bibles nor quote scripture. He is not born again, nor does he try to convert anyone. But he can take any problem in life and turn it over to his Higher Power. He is comfortable with his own kind of spirituality that allows him to handle problems without relapsing. In the past five years, Luis's mother died of cancer and his second-born son died in a car wreck. Maritza has had her own problems with relapse but through it all, Luis has remained clean, sober and incredibly at peace with himself and the world around him.

Three years after entering the methadone program, Luis got off disability and went to work as an HIV Educator, working with a community group counseling HIV clients. No one in the world would have given Luis a chance of recovery just a few years ago. Yet his recovery is a blueprint for how to do it right. If a positive attitude can keep people healthy, Luis should be around for a long time.

People like Wes and Luis keep me in this business. As sad and frustrating as addiction treatment can be, it is being a small player in the recovery of people like this that keeps me motivated.

Summary:

Detoxification or "detox" is where recovery begins. Detoxification is (def.) the medical process of removing the physiological effects of drugs and/or alcohol from the body. "Detox," however, addresses solely the physical part of addiction. Only after detoxification is completed, which comes as physical health begins to improve, can changes to thinking, attitudes and values truly begin. Even in the late stages of addiction, families, friends, medical professionals, and the addicts themselves often fail to recognize and address the parts of an addiction that impact and destroy all that the addict values.

With recovery comes changes to relationships: communication, trust, love, and respect. Family issues such as Domestic Violence are regularly found with addictions. The foundations of a relationship are destroyed by domestic violence and are important to address, but only when recovery starts to take place.

HIV and other medical conditions and their subsequent care must also be addressed with treatment, especially when there is IV (intravenous) drug use and the lifestyles that go with it.

Methadone maintenance is daily oral methadone, usually provided in a clinic setting. It is monitored with weekly counseling and random blood tests and is low-cost. It is often effective for those with large habits and can last a lifetime if necessary.

SECTION II

DISEASE AND TREATMENT

CHAPTER 3
CHANGE AND RECOVERY
FROM ADDICTIONS

This chapter examines the most common addictions and their traits. Terminology referring to *addictions* rather than *substance abuse disorders* is used in this text. The latter term, *substance abuse disorders*, is found in the Diagnostic and Statistical Manual of Mental Disorders, 5th Ed., published by the American Psychiatric Association and describes addiction as a mental health/behavioral disorder. The term *addiction* as used here describes those with a chemical dependency. However, there are repetitive, non-chemical behaviors that affect the brain's reward centers and lead to compulsive use creating non-chemical addictions such as gambling and computer addictions. They are addressed separately, later in the chapter.

Readers may find exceptions that question the definitions and characteristics of both addiction and recovery. The difficulty is that there are few hard and fast rules defining the creation of an addict, resulting in practitioners disagreeing over definitions. There is also confusion found between the symptoms of addiction and those of the mental health disorder, *obsessive-compulsive disorder* (OCD) which can be similar. *Addictions have physical, psychological, behavioral, and chemical symptoms. OCD occurs without chemical symptoms and is primarily a mental health disorder, separate from addictions. Also, addictions and OCD both affect the value system, causing behaviors that interfere with family, social and behavioral functioning. Again, OCD lacks the chemical (drug) component, which is found only with addictions. There are similarities in the etiologies (causes) of both addictions and obsessive-compulsive behaviors that also lead to confusion between the two. These are some of the factors making addictions so difficult to recognize, treat and overcome.*

We all know someone who has achieved recovery from an addiction with religion, will power, with or without professional help or despite overwhelming odds. At the same time, we all know someone who has failed miserably at recovery despite great effort and expense. There are no right or wrong ways to approach recovery. What follows is a simple understanding of addiction and a summary of what are usually the most effective methods to overcome one.

HOW CHANGE AFFECTS RECOVERY FROM ADDICTIONS

Recovery from any type of addiction requires *change.* Good intentions do not work. Every addict has made promises to himself and loved ones to change those behaviors causing all the problems. But unless substantial changes in lifestyle are made, recovery will most likely remain elusive.

Those who successfully recover from addictions make changes affecting *four areas of their lives.* These **areas of recovery** are:

*(1) **Physical Recovery**: (def.) occurs when habits and behaviors that negatively affect one's physical health and the body's interaction with its environment are improved.* For example, for some people this means getting into shape or perhaps achieving a physically challenging goal. For others it means avoiding habits that are related to or can trigger relapse. For some, it means a new goal, like a job or a return to school. *It is physical change with one's environment that leads to improved physical recovery.*

*(2) **Mental recovery**: (def.) change that occurs through an increased understanding of one's addiction and the behaviors related to that addiction. The addict becomes aware of the triggers for relapse that impact their life and develops an ability to change these behaviors over time.* For many, this means addressing related mental health factors such as depression, guilt or anxiety. It frequently requires looking at unpleasant memories of the past and

making conscious efforts to undo the damage done by their addictive behaviors.

(3) Chemical recovery: (def.) change that occurs within the brain affecting the neural responses to stressors such as pain, fear, anger or trauma. With chemical recovery, the addict develops internal strengths that no longer require seeking out a drug to face their stressors. Confidence increases as skills and maturity grow and goals for recovery become clarified.

(4) Value recovery: (def.) positive changes in the values system centered upon taking personal responsibility for one's actions. The term "spiritual recovery" is usually used by self-help programs, but this term tends to frighten people off due to the implication that it means "getting religion." Although finding God or a "higher power" may or may not occur, it is the change of one's values that often makes the difference between recovery and relapse. Value recovery may mean more emphasis on personal responsibility or a conscious attempt to be a better person. For some it means improved interactions with others, or the improvement of parenting or marital skills. Many find that developing better social skills or becoming more honest in relationships with others helps break them away from negative people and habits. Still others find that value recovery means regaining the trust of those who have been hurt by their addictive behaviors by making amends for harm they have done.

A rather simplistic but effective definition of value recovery was summed up by Luis, a former gang member and armed robber (page 42) who described it as, "Recovery is becoming the man I ought to be."

The many definitions of addiction create much of the confusion. Most definitions are found in the areas of psychology/psychiatry, where addiction is often viewed as symptomatic of compulsive behaviors or as part of a personality disorder. With this comes the belief that all addictions are the result of childhood trauma, abuse, a form of OCD, or some other type of "behavioral addiction." The medical profession muddies these waters further by putting emphasis on the physical aspects of addiction, indicating that, unless there is actual physical withdrawal, addiction does not really exist. Add religion to the picture and addiction suddenly becomes an issue of "lack of willpower" or a moral deficiency. These multiple definitions make a solid, uncomplicated understanding of addiction almost impossible.

The definition of addiction used in this text developed from something this writer heard once in a discussion. A client said, *"I have lost little due to my (addiction). I didn't lose my job, family, finances or health. My family loves me. My friends respect me. But, looking back, any instance in my life where I felt guilt or remorse, or found that I said or did something I regretted, I was high on something. I'm not a bad man, I try to do the best I can. But if I drink, I use drugs and then I start having trouble. That is what my addiction means to me...trouble because of my drinking and drug use."* That led to developing the most effective definition of addiction this writer ever heard. **(def.) If your use of a chemical of any kind, either singly or combined with others, causes a pattern of problems that are physical, mental, emotional, social, relational or other and are initiated directly by your use of that chemical, then you are an addict.**

***

By the 1980's, the treatment of addictions was evolving. Therapeutic settings were expanding and treating more than just alcoholics. Drug use had become more prevalent and drug users needed more treatment. Not that they were not always there. It is just that previously, hospitals and clinics often had trouble getting paid for treating drug addicts. So, most who were admitted for addiction treatment were alcoholics – or so it said somewhere in the diagnosis. However, by the late 1970's, we began treating the *diseases of addiction.* There was recognition that heroin addiction is different from alcoholism which is different from cocaine addiction which is different from cannabis addiction which is different from nicotine addiction. Also, it became evident that the process of addiction itself varies not only with different drugs, but with the individual's reactions to them. Some produce symptoms quickly, some over a period of years. Some people need treatment rapidly, others battle their demons for decades. Some drugs hit their victims physically, others can be used with few physical symptoms for long periods of time. Yet, addictions are all similar diseases in need of treatment.

Disease: (def.) A d*isease is a condition of abnormal vital functioning of some or all of the body's parts, systems and structures and is characterized by recognizable signs and symptoms. Diseases are attributable to heredity, infection, diet or environment. **Diseases of addiction** make permanent neuronal changes to brain systems and structures causing abnormal functioning. They are incurable – however the disease of addiction can be put into remission.*

The understanding that addictions are diseases has come a long way. In 1928, the Board of Bishops of the Methodist Church declared that drunkenness was equivalent to a lack of morals and adultery. By the 1930's the understanding was not any better when the budding psychiatric profession believed all alcoholics were latent homosexuals. During the mid-1950's, alcoholism became the first addiction to be defined as a disease rather than a moral issue. This made it easier to treat, removing some of the moral stigma from addiction. More importantly, treated like illnesses, the recovery rate of addictions began to improve.

Some people have trouble defining addictions as diseases since addicts can do some pretty vile things to support their addictions and justify their behaviors. Of course, the definition also gets manipulated, becoming an excuse for all kinds of anti-social behavior. But keep this in mind – *no one chooses an addiction.* Yes, people make bad decisions to start using addictive drugs. Yes, some people are simply no good to start with whether or not they are addicted to anything. Yes, some have underlying mental health issues that can be disguised by drug use. But those who blame their criminal behavior on drug or alcohol use are often the ones who would have done the same things stone cold sober.

It has become somewhat of a fad to present "illness" as an excuse for unhealthy behaviors from shopaholics to purveyors of child porn. We hear in defense of those who rob, rape or engage in other antisocial activity the excuse of, "My client suffers from a disease…he's addicted to (drugs, alcohol, gambling…just fill in the blank). That is why my client stole, abused or swindled." It usually works poorly as a defense and only serves to cloud the understanding of addictions by putting morality back into the picture.

Early in my career I met my first child molester. Like most, he did not look like a monster and appeared perfectly normal with a successful career, a family and kids of his own...but he liked little boys. And when he got high, he liked his neighbor's little boys a little too much. He blamed his alcohol and drug use, citing the disease of alcoholism as the reason for doing what he did. "I was in a blackout...I don't remember a thing." I have heard similar excuses from other child molesters over the years. However, being an alcoholic or addict does not create a child molester. A drug only released that monster, it did not create it. The depravity was there before a substance entered the picture. Alcohol and drugs loosen inhibitions, but they do not create the behavior.

Part of the reason for the success of self-help groups like Alcoholics Anonymous and Narcotics Anonymous is that they emphasize *personal responsibility*, part of the "value recovery" defined previously. No blaming of other people, situations or circumstances is allowed. "You own it." You are responsible for what you do...your disease may be a trigger for your bad behavior but it is not an excuse. Addictions are diseases where both the cause and the cure are in the hands of the one who suffers from them.

UNDERSTANDING THE DISEASE OF ADDICTION

Look closely at the definition of a **disease** (page 56). *Abnormal vital functioning*...this is how addicts function, not just in part, but throughout the whole of their physical, psychological and social being. Relationships, finances, recreation and other important parts of life become wrapped in and around the use of their drug of choice. Changes in health, loss of friendships and money problems become secondary to drug use. The *abnormal vital functioning* of the addict becomes the normal, everyday way of life.

The *recognizable signs and symptoms* of an addiction are identifiable by looking at a simple combination of behaviors common to all addictions: **obsession, compulsion, progression, and relapse.** (This is not to be confused with obsessive-compulsive disorder, a separate psychiatric condition.)

Obsession (def.) *is the addict's preoccupation with his drug of choice. It is what triggers his drug use, repeatedly, despite previous negative consequences and/or motivation to remain clean. It is what tells an addict that he wants or needs his drug of choice for a given reason. Obsession is instinctual, a process urging the addict to use a drug to handle something stressful.* It is NOT withdrawal, nor are there physical symptoms. Obsession is present before the physical urge to use is there. It is what makes an alcoholic think he needs a drink to relax or to be sociable or perhaps to handle a new situation. It is what makes an addict believe he needs a pill to sleep or a joint to calm down. It is the belief that says, "I function better with a nightcap (or a joint or a pill…"). *Most importantly, it occurs without physical withdrawal and often long after the previous use.*

A few years ago, I received a phone call at work informing me that my mother had died suddenly. I instantly reached into my shirt pocket where I used to keep my cigarettes. I had not smoked in 17 years. That **is** obsession – we *instinctively* seek the drug that made us feel better.

Our culture feeds into this obsession. Watch TV for more than a few minutes per day and you will see countless exhortations to take a pill when feeling down or unable to sleep, if you need to lose weight or get more energy. "Mother's little helper" comes in a capsule or a bottle. Treatment programs often find that drug users fail to address their problems, but instead they smoke, drink or somehow ingest their answer to everything. They "don't take care of business," as one of my clients once said. Have a problem at work? Light up a joint. Marital issues? Don't talk about it, spark one up or have a drink. Job on the rocks? Get high. Money problems? Snort something…a few hits and nothing else matters. Is there a fear, a pain, a problem child or are you in trouble? Is there a phobia or a loss that you have trouble handling? Take a pill. A few hits, joints or drinks and your problem does not seem so big any more. Tragically, all this does is create more dependence on unhealthy answers.

Our culture encourages this type of response. *This is a much-overlooked but very significant part of the addiction process: By taking a drug to work through your problems, you fail to find healthy solutions with your own skills. As a result, when those who are addicted attempt recovery later in life, they often have the skills and coping mechanisms of adolescents and must learn living and coping skills all over again.*

ALICE

Alice was married for 34 years when her husband died suddenly. Her family arrived on the scene and immediately encouraged her to "…have a drink…take something to relax…take a pill so you can sleep." So of course, she did.

When I met Alice, she had been under the influence of something constantly for over two years. Her detox was long and difficult. Her withdrawal from the combined effects of alcohol and sedatives was physically and mentally horrific. But this was nothing compared to the emotional loss it created. From the moment she became drug free, Alice started to grieve. She cried endlessly, experiencing the stages of grief as though her husband had died that week, not two years previously. It was only when Alice was allowed to grieve without drugs that she could finally start working through her pain and find some closure to her beloved husband's death. Incredibly, her family was angry when Alice was discharged without medications to "help" her.

MATT

Matt was a 57-year-old successful salesman with an MBA. He was also a frequent flyer at all the local detox units. He was smart, friendly and seemed as puzzled by his inability to stay sober as any of us. I sat with Matt for many hours over a stretch of about two years and could never figure out what was triggering Matt's relapses. We were all stumped. He was active in a support group, he went to church, he went to therapy, he had a nice girlfriend, nothing seemed to help. Every three to six months I found myself sitting at Matt's bedside trying to solve his puzzle. Matt was divorced for 15 years. His family was grown and he saw them regularly. He never said a bad word about his ex-wife nor his family. He made money and he had a lot of friends. He just could not stay sober despite what seemed like great motivation. A puzzle.

One afternoon, as I was about to head home, there was Matt being brought into the hospital in a wheelchair. He was too drunk to walk. He grabbed me by the arm and 20 years of pain came pouring out. "The bitch...she took my house...she turned the kids against me...left me...cheated on me..." and Matt cried.

Later, a lot of therapy later, Matt understood that he would get depressed at certain times like holidays, the anniversary dates of his marriage and divorce, the birthdays of his children. This triggered the **obsession,** the thought process that told him a joint or a drink would make things better. Although he could get through the obsession much of the time, he would occasionally return to using to "feel better...take away a little of the pain..." and this would trigger **compulsion**, and a **relapse** soon after. It had been 15 years and he was still grieving his broken heart. Only after addressing his loss without drugs or alcohol was Matt finally able to remain sober.

Like Alice, Matt fell victim to the culture that encourages using alcohol or drugs to overcome emotional pain. By doing this, the pain could not be resolved. This led to continued use and then to addiction. **Obsession...compulsion...progression...relapse**, in that order.

The second of these behaviors common to all addictions, *compulsion, is the definitive sign of physical addiction.* It marks the bodily change, the next of the "recognizable signs and symptoms" of the addict.

Nicotine is the most widely used addictive drug, so for many it provides an easy way to understand compulsion. Most of us know someone who has tried and failed to quit smoking cigarettes. The nicotine addict will fight through withdrawal using patches and pills and groups and gurus to quit smoking. Finally, he makes it. He is nicotine free.

Then one day, someone offers him a smoke. He is tired, or perhaps nervous or maybe he is in a stressful situation of some sort.

The **obsession** says, "What the hell, it's a tough day, one won't hurt." So he has one. The next day, or maybe a few days later, he thinks, "I can handle another." Soon it is two a day. "I can control it," then it is more. Within a short time, he is back visiting the guru to help him quit again. Compulsion took over the moment he made physical contact with his drug of choice. **Compulsion**: (*def.*) *Once physical contact with the drug has again been made after a period of abstinence, the body begins to subtly crave more of it. This urge becomes more powerful with time and is followed by loss of control.* Just ask anyone who has struggled to quit any addiction.

The point is, to an addict, the need for the drug is always present. His drug has in the past made him feel better, so despite previous problems, he again uses it for relief. Then he continues to use it to meet the subtle physical need for the drug. *That* is addiction. It is simple to understand: **Obsession** is the trigger – it makes us think we need or want a drug. **Compulsion** takes over once we make physical contact with the drug.

This is followed by **progression**. (*def.*) *The course of the disease becomes more prominent and severe with time. With addictions, this is observed even when there are long periods of abstinence.* Ask anyone who has repeatedly battled alcohol or nicotine. Or ask someone who has kicked an opioid addiction. Without exception, *each time a relapse occurs, it becomes harder to quit and the periods between drug use become shorter.* This is why attempts at "controlled" drug use or drinking or substituting other drugs rarely succeed for long. Whether the individual attempts to control his drug use or tries programs designed to "teach" the social use of a drug, the success is short-term at best and usually results in relapse. *This is also why the substitution of other drugs, such as using methadone to treat opioid addiction or tranquilizers to treat other narcotic addictions must be done very carefully with experienced medical care and supportive counseling.* This often can be done successfully but should be controlled and well-monitored whenever substitution is utilized.

Finally, *relapse is (def.) the recurrence of a disease after apparent recovery. It is viewed as part of the recovery process of overcoming an addiction.* Few successfully recover from addiction on their first attempt and many will relapse periodically, especially in their early attempts to quit using their drug. *Relapse provides the strongest reason for follow up treatment and ongoing support for those attempting to overcome any and all addictions.*

I must mention that this leads to a personal thorn in my side. Over the years there have been numerous programs that claim to "overcome" or "cure" addictions but never mention the need for abstinence from other addictive drugs along with continued counseling and self-help for support. Addictions are diseases that make permanent neuronal changes in the brain's chemistry and are rarely, if ever, successfully controlled. You cannot safely "teach" an alcoholic to be a social drinker nor a heroin addict to become an occasional user once they suffer from addiction. *Nor can you ever use another addictive drug safely, since the behavior will likely continue with other drugs.* Once addiction is present, one cannot learn to "use drugs occasionally" any more than a heart disease patient can learn to "just eat fatty foods occasionally" or a diabetic to, "just binge on carbohydrates occasionally." These are not safe choices and not appropriate any more than "you can just have a few drinks or shoot an occasional bag." These attempts do not work and usually lead to disaster. I have witnessed far too many suffer and die in these vain attempts to *return* to safe use. *Once you have a drug problem, you don't go home again.*

One of my clients described his struggle to quit smoking cigarettes. He struggled and quit at least 12 times. At one point, he even managed to quit for a year, only to light up once again. One of the observations he made was that *every time he relapsed, it became harder and harder to quit.* Shortly after each relapse, he was puffing away as though he had never stopped at all. On his last attempt to quit, he found himself literally praying to stay away from cigarettes. The birth of his first child was the additional motivation he needed. He is now smoke free over ten years.

Finally, as with all diseases, the symptoms of addiction come in *three stages, or levels of impairment –* **early**, **acute**, *and* **chronic**. Perhaps the only exception to this is seen with cocaine and methamphetamine addictions and powerful opioid addictions like fentanyl, where many users develop late stage or chronic symptoms very rapidly, sometimes literally overnight. We will look at these later.

Most of us when asked to picture an addict, build a minds-eye image of someone in the latest, most chronic stage of the disease. *A*

***chronic* disease** *(def.) is one which persists over a long period of time, often for the remainder of the lifetime of the individual. Addictions are chronic diseases that cannot be cured but their progress can be halted. An addict who stops using his drug is still an addict, but the disease is arrested.*

Try this – close your eyes and picture an addict. Go ahead, try it. What do you see? Someone on skid row? Someone who can no longer hold a job? Perhaps you see a relative or a friend who drank or drugged away his family. Now picture a heroin addict. What do you see? An emaciated junkie in an alley or a doorway with a needle in his arm? Remember this – no one started out that way. *The most chronic, late-stage addict was once young, with dreams and plans for the future.* Maybe that addict was once in love. Perhaps that late-stage addict who just showed up in your thoughts was a talented artist or musician. Maybe he or she is highly intelligent. (One of many surprising facts about addicts is that the average IQ of someone showing up in treatment is over 125, in the Bright-normal range of intelligence. One of my clients pointed out that you have to be intelligent to be an addict because you must be smart enough to convince yourself and others that your crazy behavior is normal.) Tragically, it seems the only time we can recognize and diagnose an addiction is in the late or chronic stages of the disease. By that time, the addict may be too far gone physically and mentally and the things he values may be too trashed for that person to recover.

Why is this important? Think of Patrick, the frightened, defrocked priest who died because no one knew how to address his drinking until he was literally dying on the job. Think of Henry, who died alone in a doorway, believing to the end that he could not be an alcoholic because he had never missed a day of work. Had their addictions been addressed at an earlier stage, they might have put their lives back together.

RECOGNIZING THE STAGES OF ADDICTION

The **early-stage** addict is hard to diagnose and harder to recognize, but the symptoms are there. (The *stages of addiction* are also called *levels of impairment*.) First however, we need to know what *not* to look for. *In early-stage addiction there are few, if any, physical problems and little noticeable withdrawal.* Early-stage addicts are usually young and able to maintain their looks, wind and stamina. They often have healthy, supportive relationships and work steadily. So what do we look for? First, there is *a pattern of regular use that, over time, eliminates other activities not involving the addictive substance.* For example, the adolescent who only hangs out with kids who smoke pot because, "everyone does it." The people who avoid parties and activities where alcohol is not served, or leave early because those who are not drinking or getting high are boring." It is those who cannot relax without a drink or a drug. It is those who have fewer and fewer friends who do not use drugs or drink.

Early-stage addicts *(def.) are those who wrap increasing amounts of their social, family and psychological supports around the use of an addictive substance.* Although they remain physically and mentally sound and appear to function normally, *they develop a pattern of regular drug or alcohol use as their lives become steadily enmeshed in the use of a drug to function.*

Look at any college campus. "Partying," getting drunk or high, is seen as normal behavior for many who are away from home and independent for the first time. They are perfect candidates to develop addictions. They are frequently lonely, often shy and lacking self-confidence. What better way to fit in than getting stoned or drunk with a bunch of other kids away from home for the first time.

I instructed an alcohol and drug education program at a local state college for about ten years. The program was aimed at students who got into some type of legal or academic trouble related to drugs and alcohol. Among students referred to the program, 70% did not return to school the following year, almost always due to excess partying. All were able to relate serious social problems that ranged from drunk driving accidents to being raped. A young girl in one of the groups pointed out that you make an easy target when you are intoxicated. This pretty, intelligent girl tearfully described being raped by an upper classman while drunk. Of the nine other girls in that group, six admitted to a similar scenario of having sex while drunk when they never intended it to happen. Does this make them addicts? No, not necessarily. But these are youth at high risk, those who have begun developing a *pattern of problems* due to their use of addictive substances.

***

As an addiction progresses, *acute*, (def.) *sharp or severe symptoms, affecting health, family and social supports,* become more noticeable. *The onset of multiple acute symptoms marks the* **acute or middle stage** *of the disease of addiction.* These symptoms include using more of the drug than you intended, indicated by becoming intoxicated when you did not intend to, overdosing or using multiple drugs. Other symptoms include social problems like assaultive behavior, blackouts (periods of time you cannot recall), or putting your drug or alcohol use ahead of something you should value, like finances, job, reputation or your family's wishes. There is a good rule of thumb. If you suspect someone has a drug or drinking problem, ask the family, especially younger siblings or children. Or ask close friends. They see the acute symptoms regularly. They often will not cover it up.

A few years ago, I sat with a man at his kitchen table for more than an hour finding myself frustrated as he rationalized and alibied his way around an arrest for domestic violence, his marital breakup and a litany of beer and marijuana-related behaviors. He minimized it all, blaming everyone else, especially his ex-wife, who also drank too much. Of course, he indicated that everything was now under control. The only break from this was when he talked in glowing terms about his 15-year-old daughter, Cindy. Cindy is an honor student, pretty and well spoken. Just as I was leaving, Cindy came home from school. Before Dad could say anything, I asked her, "Without looking at your father, please tell me truthfully what you think of your father's drinking and pot use."

Did Cindy ever grab that one! "It stinks. I'm ashamed to bring my friends home. It's ruined our lives." She started crying and stormed out of the kitchen. Bulls eye. I did not have to say anything else. Often the surest way to find out if someone has a problem is to ask the kids. They will not usually lie about it. Oh yes, Cindy's father eventually went into treatment.

***

The third and final or **chronic stage** of addiction (*def.* pg. 33) is found with *the onset of multiple late-stage symptoms, most notably, physical damage directly related to alcohol or drug use. A chronic disease shows change and progression over time.* Addictions can be both *acute*, with a rapid onset bringing on severe symptoms, and *chronic*, with slow development of symptoms over time. This is due to the differences in the strength, toxicity and physically addictive qualities of various drugs, as well as to the individual differences in tolerance for the drugs. Drug and alcohol addictions, after a sustained period of use, will produce pronounced physical damage. Some drugs produce a rapid onset of physical damage, such as the cardiac and neurological injuries seen with regular cocaine use, methamphetamines, opioids or heavy alcohol use. Addiction to these substances can be rapid with the chronic stage reached quickly. Other drugs produce a slow onset of symptoms, such as that found with regular alcohol use, marijuana use and sedative addictions. A physical examination can usually find signs of addiction via lab work, especially with liver and cardiac abnormalities.

It is in the chronic stage of addiction that physical abnormalities surface. It is also at this time when social problems, from family disruption to employment and legal issues, have been evident for a while. Sadly, it is not until the chronic stage of addiction, long after social, legal and family problems have destroyed much of a patient's life, that a diagnosis of addiction comes by way of a medical professional.

Compulsion *(def.* pg. 61*)* is a very noticeable symptom of the chronic or late stage of addiction. It is often accompanied by *out-of-control binge use that is easily triggered.* **Binge** *use (def.) is prolonged, excessive use of a drug to the elimination of other wants or needs. It usually ends with either medical or legal intervention or* *the collapse of social supports. Binge use is often followed by long periods of abstinence from the drug involved.*

WANNABET?

There are other addictions that are often seen as mental health problems, frequently as forms of Obsessive-Compulsive Behavior, rather than addictions because there is no chemical involvement. **Gambling addiction** and **computer addiction** create similar neuronal changes and behavioral characteristics as are seen in a drug addiction. They also respond to similar treatment. Since the early 1980's technology has allowed researchers to understand that *gambling and computer addiction affect the same parts of the brain, the nucleus accumbens (NAc), crucial to processing reward and reinforcement responses to addictive substances and multiple other functions. Also, they affect the striatum, a set of structures that coordinates decision making, motor control, reward perception and habit formation.* The behavioral characteristics of obsession, compulsion, progression and relapse are as evident with a gambler or a computer addict as with any other relapsing addict. *It needs to be noted again, however, that a drug addiction always has an external chemical component (a drug or alcohol), whereas gambling and computer addictions do not need these, being mainly behavioral. The chemical "component" is found in the neuronal changes in the brains of gambling and computer addicts.*

Rich grew up with the proverbial silver spoon, pampered by a wealthy family that owned a restaurant chain. Rich liked to gamble. His problem began in college with card games and sports betting. It graduated along with him and soon grew into a costly problem when Rich discovered horse racing. Rich lost as much over a few years as most of us make in a lifetime. When he showed up in my office, everyone knew he had a problem. He had embezzled a massive amount of money from his family's business and his bookies, at least three of them in three cities, had him on payment plans. He lost his car, his condominium and all relationships. Rich was scared. He was out of control and could not stop gambling. Rich worked with me and was cooperative, struggling hard for recovery and avoiding the racetrack. However, he would periodically relapse, losing wads of his father's money. This only served to destroy any trust he had built up with his family. One thing about trust, it is easy to wreck but hard to rebuild.

Rich tried different approaches. He got active with Gamblers Anonymous, took part in group and individual therapy and even made an agreement with his mother that she handle all his money. Still, every few months he would relapse. One morning, while having coffee after his group therapy meeting, Rich mentioned how he read that one of his favorite jockeys was racing locally and he confessed that he was a little tempted to go, "just to watch him." The group successfully talked him out of it, and that day Rich found the answer to his struggle.

Each morning, Rich sat at a local lunch counter for breakfast with coffee and a newspaper. That paper published the daily racing results and information on the next race card. Reading the racing forms set off the *obsession*, the mental trigger that sent Richie spiraling into relapse every few months. Once he made physical contact with his addiction by either contacting his bookie or going to the track, *compulsion* set in and he would go on a gambling binge. It took a few tries, but once Rich recognized that he had to avoid this trigger to his addiction, he was able to stop relapsing. Amazingly, one of the simplest but most significant changes he made is that now he reads a different morning newspaper. Without the racing forms to trigger his obsession, he is now able to avoid the compulsion to gamble.

Rich's gambling addiction followed the same pattern of development, from *obsession to compulsion to progression and relapse, as does a chemical addiction.* When he stopped reading the racing forms, the obsession with horse racing was no longer triggered. His compulsion to gamble then diminished and he no longer relapsed, breaking the pattern. It is important to note the similarity of a gambling addiction to a chemical addiction.

Remember, gambling is a disease that makes neuronal changes in the brain. The notable difference is that, unlike a chemical addiction, gambling has no chemical component except for those that occur within his brain when triggered by the addictive behavior. **Although there is no chemical involvement in a gambling** addiction, **Rich's vital functioning was affected when gambling triggered neuronal changes in his brain, just as a chemical addiction would do.** Again, a gambling addiction responds effectively to group and peer therapy and individual counseling, just as a drug addiction responds.

Note also the similar phenomenon seen with computer addictions, where out-of-control use essentially overtakes the life of the compulsive computer user. The similarities with a gambling addiction are striking. Research into computer addictions continues.

There is another incident with Rich that provides a lesson. When Rich came to my office, he was a recovering alcoholic for over five years. One day, driving home from work with a friend, the friend stopped and bought a six-pack of beer. Rich decided to try some alcohol-free beer. That night he drank five. The next day he bought more and drank nine. The next day he bought a case and drank eighteen. The following day he showed up in my office with the observation that he did not drink Pepsi like that. Although he did not relapse, he came close. The taste and smell of beer triggered compulsion and brought him back to his old behavior, *even without the drug alcohol* itself. At least this time, Rich recognized it before it took him down.

"IT'S JUST WEED"

Most people begin illicit drug use with marijuana. This is why it is often referred to as a "gateway drug" – it opens the gate to other addictions. This is not some great conspiracy contrived by anti-pot people. The main reason marijuana is a gateway to other drug use is its availability. It is easier to get than many other drugs, is cheaper in price and has few obvious, long-term side effects, although it does have some serious ones. Oh yeah, now it is increasingly legal. One of six adolescents who uses marijuana will move on to long-term drug use of some sort. One can easily view marijuana and alcohol as gateway drugs for much the same reason.

Marijuana is seen by many as harmless and non-addictive. It is a money-maker for states and cities and, with decriminalization, is becoming as legitimate as alcohol in some circles. Many of the chemicals in marijuana can and do have legitimate medical purposes. As of this time, it is successfully being used to control seizure disorders, reduce chronic pain and help overcome the side effects of chemotherapy. It is used to help opiate addicts kick their habit and is also, as of this time, being investigated as a treatment for autism, among other things. These are legitimate and often effective uses of marijuana and its psychoactive ingredients. *However, like many other drugs, when not used legitimately it is neither harmless nor non-addictive.*

Beginning in the early 1980's, as opioid addiction, and the use of other drugs like methamphetamines and cocaine increased, it was commonly said, even by drug counselors and medical professionals, "…what the hell, its only pot," when confronted with a marijuana dependent client. Today, with the concerted movement to legalize cannabis for recreational use, more people, especially among our young, are using it. Let us cut through the haze and take a serious look at marijuana.

I am part of the generation that popularized marijuana, the "60's" generation. For me, the dividing line was quite vivid. Graduating from high school in 1966, we all drank, smoked cigarettes and raised hell. Few if any of my classmates smoked pot. Three months after graduation, I entered college where everyone had discovered marijuana. Within a year, most of us were smoking. We all bought right into the, "It's not addictive…it's harmless," argument. Comparing the cannabis I smoked in college in 1966 to the pot available today is like comparing light beer to straight whiskey. A study in 1971 found the THC content of marijuana (tetrahydrocannabinol – the substance that gets you high) to be about 0.5 %. The marijuana taken off the streets today routinely has a THC content of approximately 20%. It has become a big market, high profit crop that has been hybridized and cultivated to a much greater potency. Another issue is Delta 9 THC. This high potency THC is linked to psychosis in many users, affecting the interplay between risk factors and mental health disorders.

Looked at another way, pot users in the early 1970's needed two or three "joints" to get high off the drug. Today, those coming into treatment routinely describe the drug as getting them stoned on a few "hits" or drags off a marijuana joint. It should also be noted that most research money goes into investigating more powerful drugs and medications. Cannabis, the dried marijuana plants containing THC, gets little money for research while more are using it, especially as it is legalized. As a result, most of the statistics and facts tend to be outdated since the strength of the psychoactive ingredients in marijuana has increased greatly over the past few years. The higher the THC content in marijuana, the more addictive and damaging it can be.

One of my friends in the mid 1960's was growing his own marijuana in the bedroom of his home. His mother thought it was part of a school project since Mick was a biology major and Mom had no idea what the plant was. He grew the plant for months and it reached a height of about 5 feet. Today, it is routine to find marijuana plants that grow up to 25 feet tall. It is indeed a different drug. There are various strengths and grades of marijuana sold in cannabis shops today, as well as pot that can be eaten or other ways ingested. As a result, pot varies in the potency and speed with which the user can be affected. (Note, marijuana "edibles" can take up to three hours before their full effect is felt. This leads to cannabis overdoses by users who think the pot they are eating is not acting fast enough, so they keep ingesting more edibles. Then they end up with panic attacks.)

I was working in an inpatient drug rehabilitation program in the late 1970's when we began regularly seeing marijuana users entering treatment. Staff could not help but notice the "non-addictive" drug was causing a lot of withdrawal symptoms. Patients kicked alcohol and other addictive drugs like opioids only to come back repeatedly with complaints that they could not stop smoking pot. *(The usual rationale was that they couldn't sleep without "one or two hits" of pot.) It must be noted that there are few, if any, effective medications for use in detoxifying from cannabis, so those kicking pot must essentially detox without medical help.* Users described a*cute abstinence syndrome of withdrawal with aggression, insomnia, anxiety with panic attacks and impaired memory.* The heavy, daily pot users were bad tempered and generally miserable. Incredibly, they would often state that they smoked pot, "…because it mellows me out." Most people do not recognize their own mood swings from long-term pot use.

Acute Abstinence Syndrome from cannabis (def.) is characterized by explosive anger, sleep problems, depression, behavioral disorders, chronic anxiety with related panic disorder and unreasonable fears. There appears to be a correlation between the amount of regular marijuana used and impairment of cognitive skills and abilities. Among the most obvious cognitive impairments are memory and impulse control problems, reduction of learning, anger control and lack of judgment. There is a strong correlation between the age at which regular use began and the subsequent impairments of skills and abilities. There is also a dissonance between the user's beliefs and the ability to practice them, i.e. belief that one is exercising good judgment while repeatedly rationalizing unhealthy or even criminal behaviors. This is seen by the user's ability to overlook unhealthy behaviors so they can justify their drug use.

One of the first and longest lasting cannabis withdrawal symptoms is a condition called *sleep pattern disturbance.* It is caused by THC interfering with sleep patterns. This is how it occurs: Those of us with a normal sleep pattern enter the first stage of sleep about seven to ten minutes after going to bed. *We then alternate in and out of various sleep stages, among these being Rapid Eye Movement or REM sleep, (def.) which comprises about 25% of our sleep time and can last up to thirty minutes per episode. It is in REM sleep that we dream. We do not usually remember these dreams unless awakened in the middle of them and quickly forget them because they do not imprint in our long-term memory.* After seven to eight hours, we awaken, refreshed.

Heavy marijuana users disrupt their sleep pattern in two ways, both of which show up when users are trying to "get clean" or stop using the drug. *First, they have trouble getting to sleep.* Many describe "counting the ceiling tiles" for hours while their minds race and, although their bodies are tired, they just cannot seem to relax and slow their thinking. Typically, they describe "just needing one hit or drag" of marijuana so they can finally get some sleep. *Once they do get to sleep however, a second problem arises. Sometime between one to three hours into the night, they awaken again. THC has disrupted their REM sleep.* As a result, many pot users describe disturbing dreams that awaken them and keep them awake. Even if they do not fully awaken, they often complain of being physically and mentally exhausted in the morning.

Put another way, when people are deprived of REM sleep, they become depressed and anxious. Studies indicate that during REM sleep, the brain processes our fears and problems through dreams which enable us to recover from the stressors of the day. Marijuana inhibits the dream process and cuts short the period in REM sleep. As a result, pot users are often less rested, more depressed and quite anxious. More importantly, they have not processed stressful issues in their everyday lives. Years of failure to process problems leads to increased diagnoses of depression and anxiety disorders and high rates of related mood disorders. These same studies indicate that sleep problems remain for six to twelve months after cessation of marijuana use. *Note: regular marijuana users (those who smoke three or more times a week) have higher rates of diagnosed anxiety and panic disorders. They voice a need to use marijuana to relax, unwind or socialize and feel "stressed" without cannabis. I find it alarming that marijuana is sometimes recommended for those suffering from chronic anxiety – the exact reason they may be suffering from anxiety in the first place.*

Another problem is *cannabinoid hyperemesis syndrome,* (def.) whereby regular users of cannabis have repeated episodes of prolonged vomiting, nausea, stomach pain and dehydration. It is found in those who use cannabis at least weekly since their teenage years, often after ten or more years of cannabis use.

It is important to note that adults who use marijuana are not as adversely affected as adolescents, with teenagers appearing to suffer more long-term, even permanent changes. The developing brains of adolescents are far more susceptible to damage to the brain's *hippocampus,* which controls short term memory and learning, and the *prefrontal cortex,* responsible for impulse control, reasoning and overall emotional stability. There are indications of I.Q. decline in heavy users as well as impaired thinking and learning. Adolescents often see their grades go from A's and B's to F's practically overnight. Behaviors change, friends are dropped and disagreeable habits like lying and stealing develop. Conversely, *those who begin using marijuana after age 25, when the brain is fully developed, exhibit fewer of these issues.*

But there is one truly scary side effect – one that all cannabis users should be aware of and that most assuredly needs more research – **Schizophrenia.**

Schizophrenia (def.) is a psychotic disorder characterized by distortion of reality, language and communication disturbances and poor social interaction as well as fragmented thoughts, perceptions and emotional functioning. Among the symptoms of schizophrenia are delusions, visual, audio and tactile hallucinations, social withdrawal, paranoid ideation and bizarre behavior. Approximately 1/3 of schizophrenics have only one episode requiring hospitalization. Another 1/3 have occasional episodes requiring hospitalization and 1/3 are institutionalized for most of their lives. Onset is usually between ages 15 and 40 years old.

There are believed to be numerous causes of schizophrenia including genetic, biochemical, psychological and social. A major genetic component shows schizophrenia running in families. But genes appear to be responsible for only part of the disease development. *A second factor, trauma, is a catalyst which might include anything from a head injury to exposure to pollutants and appears to be necessary to trigger the development of schizophrenia in genetically susceptible people. Among these traumas appears to be marijuana use at an early age. Also, recent studies find psychotic-like symptoms at a higher rate in children whose mothers used marijuana than in those whose mothers did not use.*

In treatment settings, both inpatient and outpatient, we treated *dual diagnoses* patients. These were patients with both a substance abuse and a mental health diagnosis. Whenever those admitted for a detox also carried a diagnosis of schizophrenia, *their original drug of choice, the one with which they were most likely to have begun their drug use, was marijuana.* Like everyone else, I bought into the rationale that schizophrenics use marijuana for its calmative effects. It never occurred to me that perhaps the person in front of me who has battled hallucinations for years is mentally ill because he or she has smoked pot regularly since early adolescence. *This does not mean that any teen who smokes pot will become schizophrenic. It means that marijuana use appears to put them at higher risk for this terrible mental illness.*

There have been numerous studies linking marijuana use to schizophrenia. A study in the 1980's that found a rate of schizophrenia in the general population of less than 2.0% but over 4.0% among those who used marijuana regularly. Updated research indicates that schizophrenia is three times more prevalent among pot users than non-pot users, with 42% of those having a diagnosis of schizophrenia presenting with a lifetime of cannabis use. Although the specific numbers vary, cannabis users have a rate of schizophrenia at least twice that of non-users.

Schizophrenia, classified as a *thought disorder,* is serious mental illness. Those who suffer from it usually need treatment and powerful medications for the rest of their lives. There seems to be an undeniable link between marijuana use and the onset of schizophrenia in some people. However, as of this writing, the causal link between the two has not been definitively proven. It is not known whether marijuana triggers a genetic predisposition to this mental illness or if the drug causes it without genetic involvement. But I know what I have seen. Close to 100% of those I treated with diagnoses of both an addiction and schizophrenia began heavy marijuana use in early adolescence. Also, approximately 50% of those diagnosed with cannabis use disorder have another condition such as PTSD, depression or generalized anxiety disorder.

Finally, there are other issues with cannabis that need to be addressed. As of this writing, marijuana use has been legalized for recreational use in many states and decriminalized in many others. Marijuana was historically listed as a Schedule I drug, having no medical purpose. This is wrong. New medical benefits of marijuana and its derivatives are regularly discovered with relief of pain and inflammation as well as treatment of tremors from neurological conditions discovered just within the past few years. But a significant number of negative factors arise which proponents often choose to ignore:

First, there are no cost-effective ways to determine if marijuana is affecting those driving under its influence. Alcohol impaired driving can be determined by quick, low-cost testing, such as a breathalyzer. But there are currently no laboratory determinants to indicate cannabis intoxication other than costly and time-consuming blood work. This is often not effective because THC leaves the blood within a few hours, so unless the lab work is done quickly, the result will not be accurate. Also, when a cannabis impaired driver is involved in a motor vehicle accident, there is no way to determine how recently he used, how much he used or what strength of marijuana was involved unless expensive laboratory tests are applied. As a result, lab tests are usually only done after a fatal or severe accident. These are among the problems facing law enforcement and the legal profession that will ultimately have to be addressed.

Another issue is that THC is found in breast milk. Mothers who use cannabis in pregnancy may affect the brains of their developing babies since THC is stored in the body's fatty tissues, notably the tissues of the brain. The long-term effects of this have not been well researched but, when coupled with indications of memory problems, reflex impairment and loss of motivation found in regular users of marijuana, the effects of cannabis on unborn children present factors demanding additional research. These may be factors affecting the overall mental and physical health of the children of marijuana users.

The medical profession runs into a final question: is pot safer than alcohol? The differences are often used to justify the use of cannabis, especially when it comes to which promotes more DUI arrests and/or risk of violence. Marijuana is likely less harmful than alcohol in these areas, but testing for OUI cannabis is not done extensively due to cost and time constraints. Pot also causes fewer blackout episodes, promotes less withdrawal, causes less damage and injury from impulsive behavior and has less of a link to major diseases. Alcohol, notable for links to violence and chronic illness, has fewer links than pot to chronic mental health issues like schizophrenia, and likely causes fewer lung and throat cancers. Issues specific to youth include motivational issues, DUI episodes, sleep disorders and links to the development of schizophrenia among those who start cannabis young. So, is one safer than the other? The jury is still out.

In counseling, my clients were often told that there is no such thing as a free lunch when it comes to drug and alcohol use. This addresses part of the mythology of drugs – that you can use an addictive drug safely and not pay a price somewhere in your life. Now that marijuana is becoming legal in more situations, we may be facing increased mental health problems, motor vehicle accidents and other long-term problems, and the price will have to be paid by both the user and by society.

COMIC RELIEF

One thing I am thankful for is that this business is not all sickness, death, loss and grief. Sometimes there are laughs which, although they are often at someone's expense, are necessary to keep you sane.

Most of my clients had legal problems over the years. With alcoholics, it was usually something unpleasant like domestic violence and DUI arrests. They also get into a lot of fights and generally keep the courts busy. The Chief of Probation at one of our local courts told me that his own numbers indicated that 85% of the adult criminal cases were alcohol and drug related. He added, "Mostly the goddamn drunks..." Over the years, there were numerous nuisance cases that were good for a laugh, like the guy I had who got arrested for urinating on the steps of a neighborhood church one Sunday morning during mass. He said he did not like those, "holier than thou bastards." It seems he did not like his ex-wife's attempts to get him to go to church either.

There was the pair arrested for having sex on the town common of a small local town in broad daylight after a night of drinking. It makes you wonder how they ever showed their faces – or any other part of their anatomy – in public after an arrest like that. I also met a couple who had gotten arrested for public drunkenness and inciting to riot on their wedding day. I'll bet that was quite a party. But every once in a while, I'd meet some truly memorable criminals.

Donny was in his early 20's, a quiet, soft-spoken kid who looked like an altar boy. During his intake, he told me he was on probation for the next seven years. Now, probation is regularly handed out either as a substitute for incarceration or as an "add on" after completion of a jail term so the court can keep an eye on someone. It is usually of brief duration, in part I think, because probation officers would eventually get tired of looking at the same people week after week. Seven years was unusually long.

Donny explained that he had been on a week-long Vodka binge and, running out of cash, decided to rob a restaurant. With plenty of liquid courage, Donny grabbed a knife (thankfully, he did not own a gun) and set out on his life of crime. Donny walked into a large, crowded restaurant at dinnertime. There was a line of people waiting to be seated. He cut the line and told the first person he saw, a waitress, that this was a robbery. She told him to take a seat. He did. When the police arrived, they had to wake him up. Donny said it was embarrassing to have everyone laughing at him. Donny was sentenced to seven years probation. It probably helped his case when the restaurant manager testified that they should have paid him for providing entertainment.

Another great criminal mind was Mike. Mike was a heroin addict and poly drug user who would take anything to get high and ended up dying of HIV. His career as a bank robber is truly memorable, though. Mike needed money to support two habits, his and his girlfriend's. "She was very demanding," he told me. Very dope sick too, no doubt. Mike decided to rob a bank, the Worcester branch of a local Savings and Loan. Mike did the right planning, rehearsed his actions, got his gun and ski mask ready and entered the bank. The main counter in front of the tellers had a glass partition, about a foot high, running along the top of it. Mike charged in and yelled, "This is a stick-up," and leaped over the counter ala' Bonnie and Clyde. However, his right foot caught the glass partition and Mike and the partition went crashing down. Mike said, "My ski mask was all twisted around and my gun went flying across the floor. There was broken glass everywhere. I looked through the fabric of the ski mask and they were all staring at me like I was some kind of asshole." He picked up his gun, gathered up some money and ran out to his car. He followed his plan exactly as he had rehearsed it and drove around the back of the plaza, only to find a tractor trailer blocking his way. He had to turn around and drive back in front of the bank just as the police showed up and alarms were wailing.

Somehow, Mike got away. The police eventually busted him for the bank job but could never prove it. But they have their ways of getting even. "They kept me locked up for 22 months awaiting trial. It cost me $10,000 for a lawyer. I got about $2,000 in the robbery. I'll never rob another bank again."

Mike is one of those people I miss. He bragged about his crimes the way some men brag about romantic conquests. He loved stealing and once told me that he found living, "like normal…you know, earth people…" to be boring and stealing was the only thing that excited him. A true sociopath, he had no conscience and acted on impulse, never thinking about the consequences. This way of life cost him 17 of his first 40 years behind bars. Ultimately, the lifestyle also gave him HIV and an early death.

Summary:

Addiction has multiple definitions depending upon the discipline defining it. Recovery requires lifestyle changes, not just good intentions. Those in Recovery make changes in four areas: Physical, Mental, Chemical and Values (also called "spiritual" change).

Physical Recovery: Change that occurs with habits and behaviors that affect one's physical health and the body's interaction with its environment. It is change within one's environment that can lead to improved physical recovery.

Mental Recovery: Change that occurs through an increased understanding of one's addiction and its relationship to behaviors. For most this means learning what stressors trigger relapse and addressing the behavioral factors that originally led to drug use.

Chemical Recovery: Change that occurs within the brain affecting responses to mental health stressors like fear, pain and anger. With chemical recovery the brain develops internal strengths that do not require seeking out a drug to face one's stressors.

Value Recovery: Changes and improvements in one's value system that alter things affected by drug use.

*A **disease** is a condition in which there is abnormal vital functioning of some or all of the body's parts, systems and structures and is characterized by recognizable signs and symptoms. Diseases are attributable to heredity, infection, diet or environment.*

There are multiple definitions of diseases used by various disciplines of medicine, psychiatry and the legal system. (Some of these are listed at the start of Chapter I.)

No one chooses an addiction any more than they choose to develop any other disease. Self-help is successful because it emphasizes personal improvement as well as personal responsibility for one's actions.

*There are four recognizable **signs and symptoms** of addiction: Obsession, Compulsion, Progression, Relapse:*

Obsession: The addict's preoccupation with his drug of choice. Obsession triggers drug use – it "tells" the addict that he wants or needs the drug for some reason.

Compulsion: The definitive sign of physical addiction. Once physical contact is made with the drug after a period of abstinence, the body subtly craves more of the drug.

Progression: The effects and symptoms of the disease become more prominent and severe over time. This leads to binge use.

Relapse: A return to drug use after a period of recovery. This is related to Binge use, a short duration of very heavy use usually ending with medical or legal intervention.

*Addictions, as with other diseases, have **Levels of Impairment**, also called **Stages of Development**: Early, Acute and Chronic.*

Early: A pattern of regular use that develops over time and gradually eliminates other activities not involving the addictive substance.

Acute: (also called the middle stage of development) This is marked by the onset of sharp or severe symptoms affecting health, family or social supports.

*Chronic: This has multiple symptoms, most notably physical damage directly related to the drug use. **Compulsion** is very noticeable in the Chronic Stage of an addiction, with a return to the drug characterized by binge use.*

***Gambling and computer addictions** affect the same part of the brain as opioids and are extremely addictive for many. Although there is no chemical component with these addictions, there are strong similarities to a drug addiction since the behaviors, triggers and compulsions and treatment are much the same.*

***Marijuana** is viewed as a gateway drug due to easy availability. Marijuana has medical uses and is being legitimized. Average age of first use is 14 years old. Research shows cannabis impairs those under the age of 25 due to the brain not being fully developed. Use starting after age 25 appears to cause fewer problems but use before age 25 is linked to problems including lower IQ, behavioral issues, loss of motivation and memory loss. Withdrawal (Acute Abstinence*

Syndrome) from cannabis is characterized by anger, insomnia, panic and impaired memory. Users of marijuana become depressed and anxious. Long-term users can suffer from cannabinoid hyperemesis syndrome, causing severe and chronic vomiting. The impairment of REM (Rapid Eye Movement) sleep, an important part of an individual's sleep pattern, is also linked to increased mental health complaints. This causes cannabis users to have trouble quitting the drug.

Schizophrenia, a thought disorder, is major mental illness. Research finds that 2% of the population suffers from it, but 4% of cannabis users do. Pot users have 2X the risk of developing schizophrenia than non-users. Schizophrenia develops between the ages of 15 and 40. Studies link schizophrenia to cannabis, especially among those who start using it in their teens.

Social issues have arisen with decriminalization of pot use. There are increased accidents but no way to determine an OUI with cannabis, how recently it was used or the strength of the drug. Also, cannabis can be found in breast milk, affecting unborn and infants. With memory problems, mental health issues, reflex impairment and loss of motivation, the effects of cannabis on unborn and new-born children needs further research.

CHAPTER 4
CHANGES IN THE DRUG CULTURE

After a few years of working in hospital-based treatment, I noticed that things were changing. The population was getting younger and there were more hard-core addicts looking for help. Part of this was due to increased court involvement. Jails are overcrowded and probably always will be, so sending addicts into treatment was seen not only as economical but recognized as effective at cutting down on repeat offenders. Also, those seeking treatment were getting younger because drug use was starting at an earlier age. In my first two years, I rarely saw an adolescent in treatment. By the mid-1980's, kids with drug problems were everywhere.

I must be honest here. I do not like teenagers. It is not that I do not like them personally, I just hate trying to treat them. I am not too crazy about a system that puts the label of alcoholic or addict on someone sixteen years old...labels follow you forever. I saw too many kids who got drunk and did something stupid end up in treatment with an addiction diagnosis that could keep them out of the armed services, out of public office and out of any type of employment requiring a security clearance. I also ran across one who could not get health insurance later in life because of a pre-existing condition – an addiction diagnosis received as a teenager. Hopefully, elimination of pre-existing condition clauses in insurance policies put a stop to that.

It was pointed out earlier that no one chooses to become an addict. However, we do choose actions that affect our future. Most people start making choices to use drugs, including alcohol, when they are in high school. By doing so, they start ingesting highly addictive chemicals at a time when neither their bodies nor brains are fully developed. There is often little self-control, an immature self-image and an overwhelming need to fit in. They also do not have a good understanding of consequences related to their behavior. It is tragic that our culture views kids' drug and alcohol use as a rite of passage. Immature youth make life-changing decisions to use highly addictive substances and no one takes it seriously. They make mistakes – but they do not *choose* to become addicted.

Over the years I have asked hundreds of people at what age they began using a drug – any drug including alcohol. The average age: 14 years, 2 months. (This was my own research. Hazelton, a highly respected treatment program, found the age to be between 13 and 14.) Why is this important? *If as an adult, you have managed to avoid using drugs and alcohol before the age of 21, chances are pretty good that you will never develop a problem with either. But if you start younger than that, chances are pretty good that you will have a problem.* Yet it remains a mystery why addictions are so poorly understood by the medical profession when collectively they and their effects are the nation's #1 health problem.

In 1981, I left the hospital setting to start seeing clients in the mental health clinic of a local Health Maintenance Organization (HMO). It was to their credit that they were one of the first HMO's in our area to openly address addiction. Working with this HMO meant that I now worked with people who could, and often would, remain in counseling with me for years. In the early 1980's this HMO was a small group practice plan, owned and operated by physicians who attempted to offer most of the necessary treatment. None of the physicians specialized in addiction treatment and many acknowledged knowing little about it. I was fortunate enough to be able to help implement drug and alcohol treatment and we developed a good program.

Drug and alcohol treatment in the HMO fell under the "behavioral medicine" heading, putting it under the umbrella of mental health. Once a medical detoxification was completed, treatment landed in the lap of the psychiatrist. He usually deferred to the addiction counselors, only getting involved when clients needed medication or when other medical decisions or psychiatric issues had to be addressed.

One of the first problems I encountered at the HMO was getting doctors to understand that treating a drug addict's drug addiction with addictive drugs is not a good idea. This is not a problem unique to either managed health care or to the psychiatric profession. A physician's job is to treat patients. Medical treatment is usually accomplished by either surgery or medication. Since addictions cannot be removed surgically, but they do often mimic emotional or psychiatric issues, the most well-intentioned physician is ready with his prescription pad to help his patient. Unfortunately, many medications, from mood altering drugs to sleep medications and analgesics have a high potential for addiction. Incredibly, doctors always seem to feel betrayed when the drug addicts they treat with addictive medications become addicted to their medications.

As I write this, the evening news is covering the unfortunate arrest of the daughter of a prominent politician. A pretty young woman, she has become one of millions addicted to prescription medications. This 25-year-old mother of two from a privileged background was arrested for seeking a sedative with a forged prescription. The medication she was seeking was a *benzodiazepine, (def.) part of a family of psychotropic (mind altering) medications commonly used to treat anxiety.* Initially touted as having a low potential for addiction, these medications have proven to be dangerous when administered at high dosages or to someone with an addiction. The drugs are prescribed, so many hooked on them do not realize they are addicted – until their anxiety returns and they need more and more of the drugs to feel somewhat normal.

It is a cruel irony that when attempting to withdraw from benzodiazepines a common side effect is increased anxiety, often the exact symptom that the patient sought to treat in the first place. *I must note here that this is not to imply that benzodiazepines are unsafe or unhealthy.* Short-term use of these medications with medical supervision helps most people deal safely and effectively with a multitude of emotional health issues. *The emphasis here is on short term, time-limited use of these medications, because with benzodiazepine addiction, as the body develops a tolerance to the drug, anxiety attacks can increase.* Patients soon return to their physician complaining of worsening anxiety and too often their dosage is increased. Over time, chronic, long-term users often begin to look "stoned" with glazed eyes and excessive fatigue. It should also be noted that up to 30% of fatal opioid overdoses involve concurrent use of benzodiazepines. In spite of this, patients complain of feeling terribly anxious. Most who reach this point will probably use medications for the rest of their lives, unless they find a skilled physician who can help them through a very slow and difficult detoxification while addressing their anxiety with approaches like behavior modification and psychotherapy.

BARBARA

Barbara was a high school history teacher in her mid-fifties. Unmarried, she referred to herself as an "old maid." I liked Barbara. She was not one to whine or complain and was independent, gracious and dignified with a wonderful self-deprecating humor. She hoped to travel the world and would get excited when planning to see the places she only talked about in her classroom.

Barbara saw her physician regularly. He was a classic small-town doctor who actually made house calls and knew all his patients by first name. She trusted him implicitly. When Barbara started experiencing symptoms of menopause in her late forties, the good doctor gave her Valium, a common benzodiazepine, for mild anxiety and sleep. Barbara took it for about eight years, never once altering her dosage or abusing it. Then one summer, she went on a vacation and decided, "What the heck it doesn't seem to do much anyway." So she quit. Abruptly. Addicts call it quitting "cold turkey." A few days later, Barbara was lounging in the swimming pool of a Cape Cod hotel when, for the first time in her life, she suffered a seizure. Pulled from the water, she was rushed to the only hospital on the Cape where she came close to death. Barbara had made a near-fatal mistake. Abrupt withdrawal from benzodiazepines can trigger seizures.

After returning home, Barbara dutifully went back to her physician who, after admonishing her not to get off the pills, now increased her dosage. But since her seizure, Barbara had started to experience other withdrawal symptoms like cramping and muscle spasms. And yes, her anxiety also increased. Barbara, the lady she was, did not want to ask for more medications. She instead found that a glass of wine helped her sleep. What Barbara did not know however, is that alcohol is **cross addictive** with tranquilizers (*def.*) – *both are central nervous system depressants and act similarly in the brain. If you are addicted to one sedative, you are addicted to others.* Within a short time, Barbara's drinking began to spiral out of control.

Another problem affecting Barbara was **synergism**, *(def.) a phenomenon in which two drugs taken together have a combined effect greater than the effect of either taken separately.* Alcohol and benzodiazepines are synergistic. They multiply their combined effects. It is as though three drinks and three pills do not equal six of either, but more like nine of either. The combined effects of Valium and alcohol took their toll. Barbara was found dead in bed after not showing up for school. The world lost a lovely, intelligent lady. Barbara taught school for over thirty years. She never reached retirement and never got to live her dream of travelling.

Those who find proper treatment and can detoxify from a long-term "benzo" habit pay a terrible price. Another teacher, Tom, went through some of the worst withdrawal I ever witnessed coming off fifteen years of benzodiazepine use. He was forty days in a medical detox with almost non-stop muscle spasms and cramping. He could not eat nor sleep and would go on crying jags regularly. He suffered from panic attacks for over a year after leaving the hospital. He beat the habit, but only with a lot of help from friends and his support group.

Drug habits are hard to break, especially when the dealer has M.D. after his name. Again, this statement is not meant as an indictment of the medical profession, for many an over-prescribing physician has the best of intentions. A good example is one of the psychiatrists with whom I worked who insisted on giving many of his patients a common benzodiazepine with no knowledge as to whether or not there was a history of addiction. His rationale for this was understandable but underscores the problem. He said that since many of his patients were either anxious or depressed, he figured that giving them a benzodiazepine was safe, since it is very hard to fatally overdose on them. Unfortunately, many of those patients also drank alcohol to excess, so an overdose was not only possible, it was likely.

ADDICTION AND TREATMENT EVOLVE

At the HMO where I now found myself working in the mid 1980's, the treatment of addictions was evolving. Better care was now being offered as improved policies and procedures for addressing addicted patients were developed. *But the need for treatment suddenly became more urgent with two frightening new factors, and the first came in the form of a powder – cocaine.*

When I started with the HMO, I asked my predecessor whether he had seen many cocaine users. Cocaine was beginning to explode nationally and, although I had seen a few who used it, I had not seen much in the way of addiction. Little was known about cocaine at the time. It was often viewed as only mildly-addictive, and the compulsive use of it was compared to eating a tasty snack – once you had a little you just wanted a little more. I was told that in the previous year, they had seen perhaps six or seven cocaine addicts in treatment. Within months there were six or seven per week. Within a year, most of my caseload was made up of cocaine users.

Alcoholics often drink for ten to twenty years before their problems surface. Heroin addicts can use for a substantial amount of time if there is money and a supply of the drug available to them. Those addicted to the most common drugs use for years before a problem surfaces. Cocaine and methamphetamines rewrote the script. It is not unusual to find someone seeking help for cocaine or meth dependence after only a few weeks of use. When it is smoked, a few days of use can bring people to their knees.

***

Mary was an attractive young woman who had just graduated from college three months before ending up in my office. She started work at an investment firm right after graduation. The second day on the job, Mary went to lunch with a co-worker who introduced her to her first "line" of cocaine. It made her feel great at first, more energetic and upbeat. It seemed to help her do her job better. Within a month she was using cocaine daily. Then it moved to the lady's room during coffee break. Then she used a little after work to socialize. It quickly became a financial drain. When she called me in tears one Monday, she had gone through her paycheck, emptied her savings and was severely depressed. She could not sleep without a bottle of wine to calm her and found she could not quit using cocaine. Her colleague was fired for missing work and was calling Mary trying to sell her more coke. Mary kicked her habit, but only after building up enough courage to stop taking her friend's calls.

Mary did not know that a drug dealer is not usually some shadowy figure in an alley or a hustler working the local lounge. A drug dealer is usually your friend, your neighbor, your classmate or a family member. It is the guy at the next machine or the nearby desk. He (or she) does not drive a big fancy car and is not the one smuggling kilos of drugs from another country. Drug dealers are, for the most part, chumps supporting their own habits.

I have always been amazed at the number of times clients told me how they thought they were going to make "big money" dealing cocaine, and by the early 1990's, methamphetamines. In 1995, I went through my caseload and found fourteen clients who claimed to have dealt over a million dollars worth of these drugs. Although most exaggerate, a review of their histories confirmed that they all dealt a hell of a lot of drugs. All but one of them ended up broke, sick, incarcerated or dead. The one who did not become an addict never used methamphetamines or cocaine himself.

Mario was a tall, good looking kid from Shrewsbury Street, the "Little Italy" of Worcester Massachusetts. By the time he was in his mid-twenties, he had amassed a lot of money dealing cocaine. "I had a T-Bird and a Caddy…and a girl on each arm. I had a couple of thousand dollars in my pocket at anytime. I didn't work and I had it all. Then one day, the party ended. I got busted and all my friends disappeared. I was broke. Just like that." Mario did some time in the House of Correction and went to a halfway house, where he was diagnosed with Hepatitis B and C. He cleaned up his life and was working steadily. Just before this work was published, I read of his death. Liver disease caught up with him. He was 55 years old.

Gerry was a lot like Mario, only younger. Gerry started using drugs at age 12. His mother was dying of cancer so Gerry got her some marijuana to ease the side effects of her chemotherapy. He got himself some too. His Mom died when he was 15 and Gerry was on his own. His family did not like him and left him to his own designs. He quit school and, rather than work, began to deal marijuana. He survived quite well. For a while his pot business kept him in food, new clothes and paid the rent for his mother's apartment. He brought in a succession of girlfriends to share his place and no one bothered him. Then, he too discovered cocaine. He was just 16 years old.

Gerry was seduced by the easy money. It did not take long for him to realize that, if you pay $2000 for a quantity of cocaine and "step on it" (cut it with something) you now have twice the amount you started with, or maybe three times as much if you have some good cut. Bagged into smaller amounts, it sold for about $10,000. "Pretty good week's pay…"

Gerry made a lot of money. He used cocaine in the beginning but bragged that his drug of choice was money. He stopped using coke and amassed a small fortune dealing cocaine and methamphetamines to the locals. Then one day, he got busted. "I was in Grand Central Station…I had the stuff in my backpack – two kilos of cocaine. The best stuff. I would have made a killing. I was reading the paper. I looked up and I was staring into the barrel of a "38". I heard, 'Move and I'll blow your face off.' The FBI. They busted me and I went to Danbury (Federal Prison)." Gerry laughed as he told me the next part. "The judge gave me five months…I wasn't armed and I was 18 years old so he gave me a break." Then, still smiling, Gerry said, "I can do it again…so what? If they get me, I'll go back to Danbury. It's a goddamn country club. No big deal. I'll play tennis."

I lost track of Gerry. The last time I heard from him he was moving to Florida, "…where the action is." I hope for his sake he does not end up in a Florida prison. They are not country clubs. He will not be playing tennis.

COCAINE, METHAMPHETAMINE AND THE BRAIN

I began to see significant evidence in many of my clients of *organic brain syndrome* from cocaine and soon, methamphetamine use. *A syndrome (def.) is a group of symptoms. Organic Brain Syndrome is brain damage.* Although the euphoria from methamphetamine is similar to that of cocaine, "meth" lasts longer.

There are many neurological and significant physical problems from both substances. Among these are memory loss, inability to retain new information, mood disorders, depression, paranoia, sexual dysfunction and suicidal ideation. It should also be noted that, although cocaine and methamphetamines are used in similar ways, methamphetamine causes more serious neurological illnesses. Users can stay "high" for 4-5 days with violent behavior along with paranoia sometime lasting for weeks. This creates a lethal combination of effects on both the body and the mind.

One of my "regulars" for counseling that first year was Frank, a 29-year-old cocaine addict and owner of a small construction firm. He had multiple problems from coke. He first called on a Friday afternoon for an emergency appointment, "uh…for my girlfriend." It took all of 30 seconds to figure out that he was a bigger mess than she was.

Frank agreed to meet me that following Monday at my office and I told him I would arrive early to meet with him. I was there early and of course, no Frank. About 10:00 A.M. Frank showed up. A client had just cancelled so I agreed to meet with him. I reminded him that I came in early to meet with him. He looked embarrassed and said, "I forgot what time I was supposed to be here." Then he added, "I forgot where we were supposed to meet." Frank then volunteered one more problem, "I can't even remember my own phone number."

Frank, like a lot of cocaine users, suffered damage to the part of his brain controlling *anterograde memory* (*def.*) *recall of recent events*. Without this, we lose the ability to retain new information. Put another way, without this ability you have a lot of trouble remembering. The rule of thumb regarding brain damage is that most of it is permanent and irreversible. Working previously in the inpatient detoxification unit, we used to see a lot of "wet brains," alcoholics who were severely brain damaged from years of drinking. With Frank, I met the first of many, often younger than 40 years old, suffering brain damage from cocaine or methamphetamine use.

Frank eventually got clean. I followed him for over two years. He made money, drove a new car. He was a skilled contractor and a hard worker. At one point, he had a dozen men working for him – and he always carried a note pad on which he wrote everything down. He had to. He once joked that now he could see a good movie, then watch it again a few weeks later because he had forgotten most of it. My mother used to make that same joke. Only she was seventy-eight with mild dementia. Frank was in his thirties. Oh yes, Frank's girlfriend also had a cocaine-related neurological issue. She developed a seizure disorder at age 25 while withdrawing from cocaine and will be on anticonvulsant medication for the rest of her life. She had her first seizure a year before she stopped using cocaine but kept telling herself after each incident, "It won't happen this time."

Cocaine and methamphetamine use are often accompanied by heavy drinking. Sometimes this is due to excessive partying and the alcohol use that goes with it. Other times, clients call it, "...taking the wire off," referring to the use of alcohol to reduce the "wired" feeling, the agitated nervous system caused by the drugs. In my first year at the HMO I heard a couple of emergency room physicians discussing patients with blood alcohol levels (the amount of alcohol found in each milliliter of blood) in excess of .40, which is potentially lethal. This is five times the legal limit for intoxication (.08) and the point at which people are in danger of lapsing into a coma. When the blood alcohol content gets to a level like this, respiration and pulse rate are affected and there is a significant danger that someone this intoxicated will go into respiratory arrest, or perhaps be so drunk as to pass out and choke to death in their own vomit. Most drinkers never get to this point since they pass out long before they can ingest enough alcohol to stop breathing. However, *cocaine and methamphetamine users can drink to the point of losing consciousness, snort or ingest some of the drug which immediately wakes and agitates them, and then continue to drink – far beyond the point where they would have been unconscious. This puts them at high risk for brain damage from the combined toxic effects of alcohol with methamphetamines or cocaine.*

Another nasty effect is **binge** use, the excessive use of a drug to the elimination of other needs. It is not unusual to find people entering treatment who have been using cocaine or methamphetamines for four or five days without stopping to eat or sleep. These are powerful nervous system stimulants and users can stay awake for days at a time. One part of the brain affected is the **hypothalamus,** *(def.) a walnut-sized section of the brain that sits at its base just above the spinal column. The hypothalamus controls* *appetite, body temperature and sleep as well as an assortment of other metabolic functions.* Laboratory monkeys given a choice between an unlimited supply of cocaine and food choose the cocaine until they starve to death. This effect parallels that seen with another primate, Homosapien. Methamphetamine and cocaine users often show up emaciated, paranoid and sick from chronic lack of food and sleep.

Like all drug use, cocaine and methamphetamine use has evolved over the years. At first, they were primarily snorted, then smoking them became the fashion. Injecting it was always there among the IV drug use crowd. But the search for the ultimate high never stops. A state trooper described the problem as, "Playing whack-a-mole…you no sooner stop one type of use and another one surfaces." Methamphetamine has in many circles eclipsed cocaine use. Addicts tell of methamphetamine being a lengthier high with fewer health problems than coke. This is "street wisdom" which fails to mention the speed with which the addiction develops and the multiple health issues that occur as quickly, if not more rapidly, than with cocaine.

Stevie was a short, very muscular African-American who, when I first met him, insisted that, "they" were watching him at work, in stores and were following him in his car. He heard "them" talking about him on the phone, even when it did not ring. He believed that his co-workers were watching him and his wife was talking to federal agents. Stevie had all the symptoms of paranoid schizophrenia, except that he was 39 years old with no history of mental health problems. Stevie's wife told me he had been "doing meth" daily for over two months and almost never slept.

I must confess that Stevie scared the hell out of me. He was physically very powerful and by the end of our first meeting was very suspicious of me, asking repeatedly if I worked for "the Feds." After a rather nervous call to my supervising psychiatrist, Stevie was admitted to a psychiatric unit. About ten days of good nourishment and peaceful sleep and Stevie was normal again. I followed Stevie for about two years. He bonded well with one of my colleagues and became an integral part of her group therapy. He never again used methamphetamines and never had another psychotic episode. It should be noted here that Stevie never acknowledged his drug use until his hospitalization. Had his wife not made me aware of Stevie's meth habit, he might have been placed on anti-psychotic medications since his symptoms all indicated severe mental illness. Under different circumstances, a psychiatrist might never have become aware of Stevie's drug use and Stevie's case could have had a very disastrous outcome.

Not all cocaine and methamphetamine users become paranoid. Some become extremely depressed, some anxious and some have a lot of trouble feeling much of anything. Before knowing why this occurs however, it is important to understand *how the withdrawal from cocaine and methamphetamines differs from that of other drugs.*

WITHDRAWAL
(ALCOHOL, COCAINE, OPIATES and
METHAMPHETAMINES)

When we think of withdrawal, the thought that comes to most is waking up with a hangover after a night of partying. We feel sick, a little shaky, thirsty and mildly depressed. Technically this is withdrawal, but not the serious kind. **Withdrawal** is comprised of (*def.*) *a group of symptoms related to a cellular craving for the drug we have been using.* It is not a hangover – that is gone in a day or so. Withdrawal is serious and takes much longer.

Alcohol withdrawal is characterized by mild to severe tremors, nervous system effects including accelerated heart rate, increased blood pressure and anxiety. In more severe withdrawal, there are hallucinations, seizures and *delirium tremens (def.) an acute and potentially fatal psychotic reaction with extreme agitation and frightful hallucinations.* Withdrawal from alcohol can be fatal. Alcohol withdrawal begins shortly after cessation of use. However, I have witnessed alcoholics in D.T.'s who were still highly intoxicated. If there are no hallucinations or delirium tremens, acute withdrawal symptoms come on quickly, usually last one to five days, then diminish rapidly with rest and nutrition.

Most drug withdrawals have a similar pattern of recovery - acute gastritis, agitation and depression followed by excessive sleep, then gradual physical and psychological recovery. There are significant differences among drug withdrawals however. Opiate withdrawal is rarely fatal but takes much longer with acute symptoms of cramping, nausea and other gastric symptoms that do not peak until five to seven days after cessation of use and last for two to three weeks. There is often terrible leg pain and spasms that occur during sleep causing the addict to kick spasmodically (hence the term, "kicking the habit"). Long term effects like insomnia can last for weeks or even months. Opiate withdrawal also causes emotional pain with depression and agitation lasting for weeks.

Another issue making opiate withdrawal so severe is that long-term use of opiates appears to drastically diminish the brain's ability to handle pain – any pain. This is a condition called **hyperalgesia** that includes both physical and emotional pain. Long term opiate addicts have little tolerance for discomfort. In treatment, they are notorious for drug seeking behavior, never having enough pain medications and always complaining of the worst long-term pain issues.

But amphetamines and cocaine once again rewrote the rules with the typical addict exhibiting withdrawal that is different from that of other drugs. Notably, there is often little acute physical withdrawal. The symptoms are so subtle that most do not recognize them as withdrawal. Typically, after a weekend of partying, the coke or methamphetamine user may have trouble getting to sleep but once he does, he sleeps soundly and awakens refreshed. There are usually no classic "hangover" symptoms and he goes off to his job or whatever activity keeps him busy. Within the next two or three days however, he will gradually become a little irritable and anxious. By the time he is about five days away from his last use, he is "thinking" about getting high. This is not the drug craving that is usually associated with addicts, where there is physical sickness as the body's cells seek the drug that has been withdrawn. When asked to describe a cocaine craving, users often describe it as, "a thought…that just won't leave you. It's in your head and in your gut...you want it, you can't stop thinking about it…you can't get it out of your mind. But you don't feel sick." By the time this occurs, the weekend is back and the party can begin again. The only noticeable physical symptoms are elevated blood pressure and loss of appetite. It is only when the addict decides to quit for good that he finds the need for the drug is a lot stronger than he ever imagined.

A significant difference between methamphetamine and cocaine withdrawal in that there is often more paranoia with methamphetamine users. The euphoria or "high" lasts somewhat longer, but the withdrawal can also be more long-lasting and psychiatrically dangerous.

During cocaine or methamphetamine binges, periods of use that can last for days with inadequate sleep, food and fluids, the mental health of the user often begins to head downhill. It is usually here that depression enters the picture. Approximately 12% of those withdrawing from cocaine or methamphetamines describe depression with suicidal ideation. This often accompanies unsuccessful attempts to quit the drugs as well as regrets over irrational behavior.

For some, the depression comes on suddenly, often right at the end of a binge. Carolyn was one who never thought it could happen to her.

***

Carolyn was a young professional, a lesbian with an active night life in local gay bars and clubs, very smart, pretty and intellectual. Week after week in therapy she would put up a wall of reasons as to why she was different from others and why her cocaine use was really no problem. She never drove after using, she said. She never got arrested. She accepted her sexuality and her family was okay with it too. She had a lucrative career and a nice home. Her friends were just like her, and they did not have any problems with cocaine. So how could she have a problem?

The gay and lesbian community has major problems with addictions. Estimates are that up to 37% suffer from a drug or alcohol dependency. They address many issues like "coming out" and acceptance of their own sexuality. They often live with family and societal rejection as well as relationship issues and the fear of HIV disease. Their social activities are usually centered around clubs, bars and drinking. Carolyn always fit right in. She was healthy, took part in a gay support group and even wrote for a local gay advocacy weekly. Then, one evening, after a night of partying, she broke up with her partner. Coming off a two-day cocaine binge, saddened by her breakup and withdrawing from cocaine, she found she could not sleep it away and became increasingly suicidal. On an impulse, she walked into a bar and threw herself head-first into a plate glass window.

Carolyn later told me, "God watches over fools and addicts...I was well covered." Perhaps. It is nothing short of a miracle that she is still alive...and beautiful. A heavy jacket shielded her from most of the damage. For the rest, plastic surgery worked wonders.

Carolyn explained that she had occasionally been getting depressed and was feeling angry at everything and everybody in her life. On the night of the incident, she was already depressed coming off cocaine and the breakup with her partner pushed her over the edge. She had never before been suicidal until cocaine came into her life. Drug free now over three years, Carolyn today works as a mental health professional and has not had a problem with depression since.

***

Miguel was a helpline call in the middle of the night. At the HMO, I took emergency calls whenever someone needed a detox or addiction-related services in the evening. Miguel kept me up all night.

A thin, hard working laborer, I met Miguel after his wife left him. She caught him with another woman while he was on a drug binge. He moved back to his mother's home which was shared with a kid brother in the projects of Worcester. Miguel was a methamphetamine user for about three years. Like most, he started using with friends after work and it was not long before he was using every time he got paid.

For a while, Miguel tried the "easy money" approach of dealing but found that the more money and drugs he got his hands on the more he used. He realized that he could not get ahead so he quit dealing. This was a good move. But Miguel held onto one thing from his dealing days – a gun. This was a bad move. Miguel had been depressed over the loss of his wife and had made a suicide gesture, an overdose of pills, a month before we met. I never knew about the gun until I got his call. I had seen Miguel earlier that week for an individual session and got him started with a support group. He seemed edgy and the group quickly figured out that he was, "budding," a term used to describe those who are getting ready to use. (The term "budding" stands for *building up to a drink,* a phrase first used in alcoholism recovery programs.)

I received Miguel's call about 11:00 PM. Phone calls at that hour mean the caller is either very intoxicated or in lot of trouble. Sometimes both. If they do not need hospitalization, I usually try to talk them down a little and see them in the morning. The caller will usually fall asleep, miss the morning appointment and show up a few days later, chagrined and apologetic. There was no way this was going to happen with Miguel though. His first words were, "I have a gun...I'm going to die." It was a long night.

I cannot recall many details of the conversation. Miguel cried a lot and he was very angry. He hung up on me once but I called him back. Because he had made a recent suicide attempt, I did not feel safe telling him to see me in the morning. Miguel mentioned that his kid brother would be home later so I decided it would be safer to keep him occupied until his brother got home, also hoping he would sober up a little while we talked. Not only did that fail to happen, he got more agitated as the conversation went along. Miguel talked about his wife and his regret for having cheated. I heard all about his former girlfriend, his child, a lot of women he would usually view as conquests, although tonight he viewed them as losses.

At one point, Miguel's anguish built up and he banged hard on the wall next to him. The first time he did that I thought he shot himself and screamed into the phone. He would later remind me of that and thought it was pretty funny. We talked about his drug use at length. He knew, as does everyone who finds himself losing control, that the stuff was killing him. In his intoxicated, hysterical state, he fought with his own demons. I listened with an eerie fascination as he personified the drug, alternately talking to me, then to the drug and at times it sounded as though the drug itself was talking. "It makes you feel better, it gets you laid...you ain't nothing without it..." Then he would talk of "never being anything, losing it all..." because of methamphetamines and how he wanted to die because he could not quit.

By the end of the night, it was hard to say who was more exhausted, Miguel or me. Sometime after 3:00 A.M., Miguel's brother came home. We spoke for a few moments and Miguel was on his way to the E.R. Miguel had never been suicidal before this and has never again had these thoughts and impulses since being drug fee.

A quick aside: The next morning, with Miguel safely tucked into the psych ward for a detox, I went to work with virtually no sleep. My first client showed up drunk, swinging a steak knife in one hand and a beer in the other. She certainly impressed those in the waiting room. I was in no mood for Linda's bullshit. I took her knife away and screamed at her, calling her an asshole. That was not very professional. She went to detox, I went home and got some sleep.

The toxic side effects of cocaine and methamphetamines coupled with inadequate food and sleep triggers the paranoid, suspicious behavior found in addicts. They tell stories of hiding behind shuttered and locked windows, in cellars and closets and describe irrational suspicions of friends, co-workers and companions. In the mid 1980's a Massachusetts State Trooper was shot and killed by four drug suspects after a routine traffic stop. That evening, there was a door-to-door search for suspects in a nearby neighborhood where they lived. One of my clients told me about sitting in his cellar that night with two kilos of cocaine and a loaded automatic weapon while the police went house to house. My client said, "If the police showed up at my door that night, I'd have killed them. Thank God they didn't." Yes, thank God.

THEY DON'T WASTE HEARTS

Cocaine, methamphetamine, and other forms of "speed" or "uppers" have devastating effects that go far beyond mental health issues. Even doses that appear to be harmless can cause sudden death through cardiac problems. Users develop chronic high blood pressure, seizure disorders, neurological impairments as well as heart and kidney damage. In addition, there is a litany of problems associated with exposure to violence, sexually transmitted diseases and impulsive behavior.

One of my clients was excited about her sister's upcoming wedding. She was going to be the maid of honor. When the big day came, her sister suffered a stroke while "doing lines" with other members of the wedding party. The happiest day of her life was ruined. My client blamed herself for having introduced her sister to cocaine years before.

Seeing so much physical damage from drug use changed my attitude. As counselors, we are taught to detach our personal emotions from those of our clients, no matter how horrible or desperate their problems appear. This keeps us from letting our feelings become enmeshed with those of our clients. Keeping our emotions in check protects us from getting overwhelmed or "burnt out" and enables us to view our client's problems more objectively and thus do a better job treating them. But with the 1990's came an increase in drug use that challenged my ability to detach from the pain before me. Where I once found it easy to let go of the terrible losses inflicted upon my clients by drugs, I now found myself more empathetic to their pain, losses and fears. In the first five years of working with cocaine and methamphetamine users I saw six patients die from heart attacks. The oldest was forty-one. Two were listed for heart transplants but neither made it. They both returned to drug use even though they knew their heart muscle was badly damaged. At least 15 others had cardiac issues or strokes leading to hospitalizations.

I received a consult (a referral) to see a 21-year-old girl at a local hospital. She had gone into cardiac arrest while doing cocaine. When I arrived, I found myself looking at a pale, delicate child, a mere waif, hooked up to monitors and IV's. She was tiny and looked like the frightened little girl that she was. Her parents lived about three hours away and arrived just before I got there. Her mother was crying and her father was sitting at her bedside stroking her forehead. He too was crying and shaking. All I could make out was, "My baby….my little girl." She was their only child.

I felt embarrassed being in her room. I did not belong there intruding on their private tragedy. Besides, she was far too weak to talk so I quickly left. I spoke to the cardiologist who gave me some of the medical details, essentially saying that her heart was severely damaged and she would probably die soon. I asked him about treatment, medication and therapy. He said that all of this would be administered if she stabilized. Then I asked him about a possible transplant, since she was so young.

"She won't get a transplant. She probably won't last that long. Anyway, she's an active drug user. We don't waste hearts on them."

Perhaps my own personal defenses kicked in about that time, for I have blocked her name from my memory and cannot recall what eventually happened to her. But I do remember that she affected me greatly. It was early enough in my career that, for the first time, I felt very sad and could not detach my feelings. It is not that the pain poured out in my office had never before affected me, for I always empathized with clients. Perhaps it was because she was so young, so delicate or because she was somebody's only beloved child. Maybe it was her eyes – so big, dark and terrified. That morning, I went back to my office, cancelled my appointments and closed the door. I needed to be alone. Perhaps it is best that I do not know what happened to that child and her family.

COCAINE, METHAMPHETAMINES AND SEXUALITY

Whelan was an engineer with a software company. He made excellent money, owned a new home, had a lovely wife and a twelve-year old son. I never learned how he got introduced to cocaine, only that by the time he met me, cocaine had infected every facet of his existence. There was no longer a social life nor family life. The initial thrill of doing lines with a few friends had given way to snorting lines by himself, locked in his basement watching pornographic movies and masturbating compulsively. This behavior is not uncommon among cocaine and amphetamine users. By damaging the brain's **hypothalamus**, which controls sexual drive and behavior, users do not just lose sexual inhibitions, they lose the ability for normal sexual functioning. Whelan told me, during his brief recovery, "I used to be able to have sex all night, now I just can't have sex without cocaine."

About this time another client drew an excellent metaphor for understanding cocaine addiction. He said, "Take a nasty itch on your arm…like poison ivy. At first it feels good to scratch it. Soon, you scratch too much and this makes the itch worse…so you have to scratch more. It briefly feels better, but the more you scratch, the more it itches and eventually, you can't scratch anymore because it hurts too much. But you can't stop scratching because the flesh is painful and irritated. That's how cocaine works, except the need to do cocaine is the itch and the drug does the scratching. And it is your brain that becomes painful and irritated."

That analogy also explains how cocaine, methamphetamines and similar drugs affect sexuality. At first, the drug makes you feel incredibly sexy. It makes sex seem so much better that you want to do the drug whenever you have sex. Soon, you start to need the drug to have sex. Before long, you cannot have sex at all unless it is with the drug. Eventually, you can't have sex. It is not a loss of the ability to function. *It is a change, damage actually, to the areas of the brain that control specific metabolic systems and leads to disruption of the sex drive.* Men suffer from impotence and women from anorgasmia. This is why many get into pornography. They are seeking something to stimulate a diminishing sex drive. This is where Whelan was when I entered the picture.

I do not pretend to understand what happens in the mind of an addict who has become impotent from cocaine or a similar drug. Whelan described his sex drive as being normal. He said he loved his wife but, after a few minutes of lame excuses why he no longer made love to her, he admitted that his sex drive was almost gone and that he could barely perform sexually. His sex drive was only present when he did cocaine. He also said he had lost the ability to care about this. I pursued issues with Whelan's marriage, his son and his health. His answer to most of these inquiries was a simple, "It doesn't matter anymore. I just don't care."

A few weeks after our initial meeting, Whelan was rushed to the hospital suffering from a "cardiac incident" while doing cocaine in his basement. During his rehabilitation period, he was forcibly drug free and promised his physician, his family, his son and me that he would never again touch the drug. He meant it, for a heart attack gets your attention. Whelan made amends to his wife and his son and contacted his minister. He even returned to church the week he left the hospital. Less than a month later however, his wife found him in the basement doing lines of coke. A few months after that, he was dead.

Whelan's story provides an understanding of how cocaine and methamphetamines affect the brain's control centers. *Although these drugs affect the entire organ, they primarily impact the most essential parts of the brain, the areas controlling our appetite, our heartbeat and breathing, our feelings of well-being, our "fight or flight" response to fear and our sexuality.* These are not the advanced areas of the brain controlling our cognition, intellect and emotional status. Cocaine and methamphetamines do most of their work in the innermost areas, those controlling our involuntary functions (those controlled by the body's systems and independent of our will), and semi–voluntary functions (those where there is some control but most control is independent of our will), and our basic survival responses. These are found in all animals, not just primates. These are the areas damaged by cocaine and methamphetamines.

When drugs like cocaine and methamphetamines are first used, the drug stimulates these areas and users feel strong, confident and sexy. Addicts often tell of initially using them because it made them feel, "on top of the world…like I could do anything." After repeated use however, they need more of the drug to achieve those same feelings. Soon, they begin to feel frightened, anxious and suspicious of everyone. They lose the confidence and fearlessness they initially sought and become paranoid. One of the complaints often heard, much as I heard from Whelan, is, "I just don't care about anything. Nothing excites me." This is a condition called ***anhedonia***, *(def.) the inability to feel emotional stimuli, especially pleasant or happy emotions*. During this period there is an increased risk of heart attack or stroke as the damaging effects of prolonged elevated heartbeat and blood pressure take their toll.

The client who drew the previous analogy between cocaine and an itch was Gary, a 27- year-old engineer. He was married to "a fox" to use his own description of her beauty. She was too. Gary had used cocaine for about six years. For a while, he made a lot of money dealing the drug and enjoyed an expansive lifestyle. He paid the price physically though and became impotent from cocaine. After Gary first disclosed this problem he said, "It doesn't bother me that

I can't function (sexually) but it's beginning to bother my wife." I asked him to discuss this more, pointing out the obvious. "What do you mean, it doesn't bother you? You are married to a beautiful woman whom you love and you have had sex twice in a year. You are here as a result of this and you say it doesn't bother you?" Gary looked at me for a long, silent moment, carefully composing his thoughts. "You don't understand. It's not that I don't care about sex or that I don't love my wife. It's just that I don't care that I don't care." Like Whelan, *Gary too was describing anhedonia. In the brain of virtually all chronic cocaine and methamphetamine user I have ever met, there is a low-level depression caused by damage to the organ that once held the human feelings of affection and caring, that provided confidence, self-respect and inner strength. These are all the things that make us human. That is what methamphetamines and cocaine damage. And not only do you feel nothing, you cannot even care that you feel nothing.*

TRIGGERS

All drugs of abuse have *cues* or *triggers* which set people on the road to using drugs. A *trigger (def.) is a substance, object or agent that initiates or stimulates drug use..* At AdCare back in the early 1980's I used to hear alcoholics regularly complaining that every time they looked out the window at the end of the hallway, they had to look at a liquor store. So many complained about it making them want to drink that we had to discuss it in group therapy. It usually is not that obvious, but many things create stressors that can trigger drinking or drug using episodes, such as anxiety, loss, physical or emotional pain or financial problems to name a few. Among heroin users, one of the worst triggers is any physical symptom that mimics withdrawal. I remember thinking how strange it sounded to hear a man in group therapy say, "I woke up with a runny nose….so I had to get high." It did not sound strange to anyone in the group, though. They all knew that trigger because when withdrawing from heroin, your nose runs incessantly.

Drugs like cocaine and methamphetamines have many triggers in common. However, there are **three triggers** that must be addressed if someone is going to overcome any drug or alcohol addiction, whether it be an "upper," a "downer," a hallucinogen or other commonly abused drug. *For that matter, avoidance of these triggers is vital for recovery from all addictions.* **The first of these is *alcohol use*.** It can safely be said that every recovering addict should stay clear of alcohol. Most people who use "speed" or "uppers" will either drink alcohol with it, prior to getting it or immediately after using it. Anytime they drink alcohol, there is a distinct danger that their brain will unconsciously associate the sensation with cocaine or other "speed" use and a relapse will be triggered. Also, alcohol reduces inhibitions and impairs judgment. So if someone says, "Hey, let's go get high," their defenses are gone. *When a cocaine or methamphetamine user drinks alcohol, he is in dangerous territory.*

Among heroin users as well as those who use "downers" such as tranquilizers, narcotics or sedatives, we see a similar phenomenon. Addicts in recovery who begin to use alcohol are at extremely high risk for developing alcoholism. *This is an example of cross-addiction, (def.) those addicted to one sedative are addicted to all others.* Those addicted to heroin, a *nervous system sedative, (one that produces a calming or tranquilizing effect on the brain),* are cross addicted to alcohol, another sedative. *This occurs whether or not they have previously used alcohol.*

A second trigger is *money*. I heard many addicts say, "A twenty-dollar bill isn't twenty dollars, it's a rock (or a bag)." Relapses occur so often on pay day that, as part of behavior modification, many clients have their paycheck sent to a trusted family member or neutral party and doled out in small amounts so they do not get triggered by the cash. Two of my clients, a pair who could not be more opposite, found common ground addressing this trigger.

Gerry is a classic redneck. Before it became politically incorrect to do so, he drove a pickup truck with a confederate flag in the rear window. He was uneducated and unrefined, bigoted and opinionated. In another era, he would have been in the KKK. I used to love sitting him between clients of different races in group therapy. I knew it pissed him off but it just seemed like the thing to do if Gerry was going to grow up. Anyway, I secretly loved the entertainment. This nearly backfired one evening when Malcolm, a very large, very successful African-American pointed out to Gerry that it did not bother him to buy drugs from minorities if they were selling cocaine. They nearly came to blows and I had to consider the wisdom of keeping them together in the same group. But sometime things happen for a reason.

Shortly after his dustup with Malcolm, I found Gerry waiting for me at my office when I arrived one morning. He had no appointment but, from his look and smell, he had been on a cocaine binge from hell. It was Friday, the day after his payday. Gerry claimed that yesterday, as well as the previous two Thursdays, he received his paycheck and, other than a few sparse details, could remember nothing until he arrived at his cocaine dealer's house. He was describing a *blackout, (def.) a period of time in which a person under the influence of a drug appears to function normally but cannot remember some or all of his actions.* The only difference here was that what he was describing occurred prior to his using anything at the time. He had not been drinking when the blackout-like behavior occurred, nor had he used anything else that day. His cocaine use had become so chronic that money now became only a trigger to further cocaine use. He sobbed, telling me that he could not remember driving, he just remembered arriving at the dealer's house. He said that all day he had been thinking about getting high and could barely function at work. Gerry once described getting high with an almost sexual obsession, "…an orgasm in every cell." Now though, the fun, the excitement, the "turn on" had stopped. To make matters worse, Gerry feared that this would never stop happening. He was afraid to go home, saying his wife would never believe him nor forgive him and would have his bags packed on the front porch. His life was totally out of control.

While we talked, Malcolm came into the waiting room, awaiting his own appointment with me. As Gerry and I walked out of my office, Gerry took one look at Malcolm and broke down sobbing. This took Malcolm by surprise and in a minute the three of us were in my office talking and looking for answers.

About a week before, I had to separate these two men to keep them from hurting each other. As they talked in my office this day, I watched as Malcolm fully identified with Gerry's pain. He too was fighting the same demon, and I must admit I was amazed when Malcolm offered to drive Gerry home and stay with him for a while.

I had no idea how this was going to work out. I had planned to meet Gerry's wife later that day to try to diffuse the situation. Instead, Malcolm went home with Gerry, spent the entire day with Gerry and his wife and even bought them lunch. Gerry began going to AA meetings the next day, with Malcolm driving. Gerry followed the group's suggestion that he have his wife pick up his paycheck and dole out money for his lunch. It worked - far better than I could have dreamed.

Despite their differences, Malcolm identified with Gerry because they had the same triggers. Malcolm was financially well off by most standards. He drove a new Mercedes, owned a business and wanted for little. He was liberal, friendly and outgoing. As time went on in the group, Malcolm would jokingly race bait Gerry. He viewed Gerry with amusement but a compassion that likely saved Gerry's life. "Hey Gerry, you look patriotic. Red neck, white socks, blue ribbon beer." Gerry would toss a few wisecracks back at him and everyone would laugh.

One Tuesday night, Malcolm did not show up for group. He had started on a cocaine binge that nearly killed him. He did not stop using for a month. His wife left him and one of his sons ran away and was picked up with another teenager in New Jersey. Malcolm emptied a bank account and maxed out two credit cards before he was stopped. Malcolm's binge was stopped by Gerry, who went looking for Malcolm and found him walking out of a crack house. I was upset with Gerry for putting himself in that position because just being in that neighborhood was a powerful trigger. But Gerry found Malcolm and, unannounced, was in my office with him the following morning.

It was obvious from talking with Malcolm that he was not able to stop on his own. He had sold his year-old Mercedes for a thousand dollars, was sharing a house with prostitutes and drug dealers and was hanging around with a particularly vicious street gang. He told me later that he was also carrying a gun. It took a few phone calls but Malcolm was soon on the way to an inpatient program in another state. Gerry drove him there.

As they talked on their way to the treatment program, Gerry identified one of Malcolm's triggers. It seems Malcolm would drive around Worcester listening to rap music. He would get excited and tap rhythmically on his steering wheel and the next thing he knew he would be in the old neighborhoods where he used to buy crack. One day, while stopped at a traffic light, to his left was an old "friend," a dealer he had known from previous use. "It was like I never stopped using. Suddenly, he was in my window and I was buying some rock. It was as easy as that."

Gerry and Malcolm spent a lot of time together when Malcolm returned to group. Gerry suggested that the rap music also needed to go. He took great pleasure in adding, "That shit would drive me over the edge too." But the real change came via Gerry. Since his own relapse, Gerry's wife handled all his money. That was easy for him since he did not have much money anyway. Gerry suggested that Malcolm also add this to his plan for recovery. This relapse had cost Malcolm about $50,000. From that time on, his wife handled his money. He drove around in his Mercedes (he got it back from a drug dealer a little beat up but still a nice car) with a brown bag lunch and $5.00 per day. He said it worked. "No money…it's a big trigger I don't have to deal with any more."

For at least five years, Malcolm has carried no credit cards, no ATM card, and little cash. He and Gerry have remained friends, each crediting the other for saving his life.

The third trigger, after alcohol and money, is *people*. It is a trigger common to most addictions. Drug use is not just a habit, it is a lifestyle. It is how we socialize, how we express our feelings and how we become part of a group. It is how we meet the opposite sex. The longer we use a drug, the more likely it is that most of the people we associate with are also drug users. This is whether drinking in a neighborhood pub or getting high in a crack house. *Drug addiction is comprised not only of the chemical we use but the people we use it with and the circumstances around that use.*

If everyone living in your neighborhood, family or apartment building is a drug user and you need to avoid these people to stay drug free, you have a major problem. *People* become the most difficult trigger because few addicts have either the will or the finances to move away from their friends, family and neighborhood – even if it is killing them.

STRIKE THREE

Joey B. wanted to be a professional baseball umpire. He worked his way into sandlot ball, umpiring local minor league games. Originally from Idaho, he had migrated to New England in pursuit of his dream. He once said, "In Idaho no one was using cocaine, at least not in my town. But there is not much baseball either. I have no future there." Unfortunately, his future got detoured in Worcester when he got introduced to crack cocaine.

I watched Joey kick his cocaine dependence five times in less than two years. After each struggle, he would run into a "friend" who had some crack and then relapse. Once, he even hopped a greyhound bus and went across the country. Reaching Los Angeles, he got some work, saved up enough to come home and arrived back in Worcester, completely detoxified and healthy. He was not in town two days before he ran into another friend and more crack.

Shortly after his last detox, Joey showed up at my office unannounced. "I want to thank you for trying to help me…but I have to get out of here. I used again this weekend. I can't stay away from the shit. I walk out my door and there is a dealer on every corner. I can't go within a few feet of my room where there is not someone with a rock." Joey showed me his ticket out of town. He was heading back to Idaho. He could not stay clean in Worcester, "I have no future here."

Joey was one of the lucky ones. He was able to leave his triggers behind him. He had neither a girlfriend nor a career, did not own a house nor have a family to keep him from escaping "a place where everybody uses." As I think of Joey, I wonder how anyone living in the projects of a city, or how someone living with an actively using addict can beat an addiction when it seems that everyone around them is using or dealing.

A RATIONAL EXPLANATION:
IT WOULDN'T LET ME GO

Many drugs, notably marijuana, crack cocaine and methamphetamines are smoked. Although the drug is the same whether smoked, snorted or injected, smoking sends it to the brain most rapidly and with the most purity. It provides an instant euphoria described by many users as *instant addiction.* I first laughed when I heard the words, "instant addiction," believing that the neurological changes caused by drugs take time to develop. I do not laugh about it anymore. My first two crack cocaine addicts nearly drove me from the business. I honestly thought, "If they're all like this, I'm outta here." I seriously considered changing my career.

Mark was seventeen, tall and skinny, chasing girls and fighting acne. He was captain of his high school basketball team, athletic and well liked. His Dad loved him with the special devotion of a single parent. Mark's mother died when Mark was a toddler, so he and his father were very close. Dad never remarried and devoted his life and energies to his son Mark.

As Mark finished his junior year of high school, he went to a party with some friends who had just graduated. It was the end of June. At the party, Mark was introduced to crack cocaine. Ten weeks later, Mark's father went away on a business trip for three days. When he returned, Mark had sold much of the furniture in the house to buy cocaine. Incredibly, his father noticed nothing amiss earlier that summer, noting only that Mark had lost some weight.

Mark's dad immediately called the police. The local police sergeant was also a family friend. Mark explained to the sergeant, very rationally, that he had sold everything to buy crack. He told the police where he got it and provided the names and locations of everyone involved, including the drug dealers. The next day, the dealer was arrested and most of the stolen goods were recovered. Later, when everyone was bailed out, the dealer and a couple of his friends were seen in town looking for Mark.

This is where I entered the story. Mark's father brought him to the clinic and I interviewed him. He was polite and rational but had no explanation as to why he did this except to say, "When I smoke coke...well, I just have to do it. It won't let you go." He described a wonderful relationship with his father and indicated no problems, psychiatric or otherwise. I saw no reason to hospitalize him, so he was sent home with a mild anti-depressant and a follow-up appointment.

That night, while his father was taking a shower, Mark grabbed Dad's car keys and wallet and drove off – heading back to the same Worcester neighborhood to find the same people he had just turned in to the police. I received a panic-stricken call from his father who justifiably feared for his son's life. I did not know what to tell him except to suggest the he contact the police sergeant and try looking for Mark in Worcester. Later that evening, he and the sergeant found Mark on Murray Avenue, at that time a less-than-safe street for a kid from the suburbs. Around 2:00 A.M. I arranged for Mark to be placed in the psychiatric unit until something could be done. At least it got him off the street.

The next day, Sunday morning, I paid a visit to Mark in the psychiatric unit of St. Vincent Hospital of Worcester. I have always found that locked wards fit as many of the "cuckoo's nest" stereotypes as you can conjure up, with mumbling schizophrenics watching your every move to sedated zombies pacing the floor. A psychiatric unit is a cold and uninviting place no matter how pretty it is painted or how professional and caring the staff may be.

When I was brought to Mark's room, he was laying on top of his bed covers staring blankly at the ceiling. His feet hung over the end of the bed and his sneakers were without laces – a precaution so he would not hurt himself. He was in street clothes, sweats and jeans. He looked like any other kid. So normal.

I asked Mark to relate the previous day's actions and he did, as politely as before. Pushing him a little, I asked him if he was aware of how much he had frightened his father. He knew this and seemed truly remorseful, telling me that he never wanted to hurt his father. I then asked him why he took the money and went looking for the same people he had just "ratted out" to the police a couple of days before. I asked, "Don't you realize that these people will kill you if they find you?"

Mark sat up and looked straight at me. "Yes, I know. One of them even brags about killing someone in Florida. But you don't understand. It didn't matter...I had to do it. I needed a rock. Cocaine doesn't let you go." I had no answer to that except to refer Mark to an out-of-state program for extended care.

It needs to be pointed out here that Mark, like all of those I have seen in treatment for crack cocaine or methamphetamine addiction, outwardly exhibited little or no withdrawal – no shakes, sweats, cramping, nausea nor anything we normally associate with coming off a drug – he simply could not control his need to use the drug once that compulsion was triggered.

Mark was later discharged from St. Vincent's and sent to a long-term program. His father sold the family business and they moved out of state. When I last spoke to his father, Mark was doing well, away from the triggers and living in a whole new environment. Again, I must wonder what options were left for this family if they were not financially secure enough to be able to pull up roots and move halfway across the country. What terrible things would have happened if they could not move away?

The week I met Mark, I also met Cindi, a twenty-year-old single mother with a cocaine and methamphetamine habit. She lived on the top floor of a three-decker in downtown Fitchburg, Massachusetts with her five-month-old son. Cindi had separated from her baby's father due to her drug use. One afternoon, Cindi put the baby down for his nap and went across the street to her dealer's house to buy a "half" – a half gram of cocaine powder which she planned on snorting. When she got there, her dealer had just cooked up some methamphetamine for smoking and was ready to party. Cindi started smoking and did not return to her apartment for three days.

Perhaps someone or something was watching over the baby that day. Around 8:00 P.M. a friend showed up for a visit. Cindi was nowhere to be found and the baby was screaming, hungry and filthy. The police were called and Cindi was later arrested and charged with felony abandonment and endangering a child.

When I met Cindi, she had just completed seven months in a halfway house. She lost custody of her son but spent a lot of time working to overcome her addiction. She had become active in self-help and developed a solid support system. She never missed her appointments and was as cooperative as any clinician could hope for. But the drug is powerful. One day, Cindi simply vanished.

It is not Cindi's actions that I remember most, it is her words – words voiced the first day I met her. She said, "I love my son and I am a good mother despite what I did. But you don't understand…I knew my baby was alone, hungry…but the (meth) pipe…it wouldn't let me go."

Cindi's words echoed those of Mark who claimed his crack use, "…wouldn't let me go." I would hear that refrain from dozens of drug smokers over the next few years.

***

Cocaine hydrochloride is derived from the leaves of the coca plant, a shrub native to parts of South America. It is processed into a white crystalline powder or used in a solution as a mild topical anesthetic. The native people who cultivate it chew the raw leaves of the coca plant for extra energy. Historically, in the late 19th century, it was touted as a harmless pick-me-up and added to many medicines and other elixirs, the most famous among these being the original Coca Cola. It was viewed as non-addictive by the medical community until anecdotal evidence of its addictive potential grew to such an extent that cocaine was finally labeled a *Schedule II Drug, ("…a strong potential for addiction but has a legitimate medical use.") In the brain, cocaine, (def.) affects the reward circuits and dopamine levels with heavy use causing negative affects upon mood and emotions. It reduces the re-uptake of dopamine (the return to a normal level), leading to depression. Long term use is linked to psychosis, paranoia, anxiety disorders and violent behavior as well as chronic headaches, strokes and seizures.*

Notable among its early proponents was Sigmund Freud, the father of psychotherapy. I met numerous clients who used this as an excuse when they rationalized its use. I had a physician tell me that he thought it should be legalized, joking, "…if it was safe enough for Old Sigmund, it should be legal." After treating a few cocaine addicts though, Freud was singing a different tune. What proponents fail to say – and perhaps choose not to know – is that Freud lost a good friend to a cocaine overdose and, from that time until the end of his life, he derided cocaine use and spoke of it as the dangerous drug that it is.

***

Methamphetamine (def.) is a synthetic amphetamine which, like cocaine, is also a Schedule II Drug. It is a strong nervous system stimulant mainly used as a "recreational" drug. It was initially developed as a treatment for Attention-Deficit Disorder. It has a high potential for abuse and today is rarely used for ADD due to the availability of safer drug alternatives. A form of "speed," it is a neurotoxin, (harmful to nerve tissue) and is often called "ice or crystal."

Methamphetamine is similar to cocaine in behavioral and observable effects. However, cocaine has a half-life (a point in time in which 50% is gone from the body) of about one hour. Methamphetamine has a half life of about 12 hours. As a result, "Meth" remains in the body – and subsequently in the brain's synapses – much longer, leading to neurotoxicity. This long half-life is one of the appealing aspects of methamphetamines for drug users. There are few medications for effectively treating a "meth" addiction. Long-term use of this drug leads to problems with attention, short term memory and judgement. The hippocampus, a brain structure providing the ability to remember and learn, and the striatum, a structure crucial to movement and concentration are impacted by meth. The parietal cortex, important for non-verbal learning, and the frontal and prefrontal cortex, crucial to cognition, reasoning, complex attention, problem solving and impulse control are damaged further by methamphetamines.

***

I was walking down my driveway that weekend after closing the cases on Cindi and Mark. As stated previously, I was honestly questioning whether I should remain in this line of work. Crack cocaine and methamphetamine users were the scariest, most unreasonable clients I ever met. An addict who becomes a criminal to support his/her habit can be understood, for withdrawal from drugs can be overpowering. They commit crimes to pay for their drugs and can become violent or abusive when under the influence. But there is an irrationality evident in crack and meth users who jeopardize life, family and health to use the drug almost before they have had time to become addicted. A drug counselor will soon realize that this behavior reflects the neurological changes that make addiction a disease. No amount of motivation, not Mark's love of his father nor fear for his own life; not Cindi's newborn child nor months in a rehabilitation program could halt their addiction. *They knew how devastating it was but did not appear to be able to do anything about it.* This is what troubled me that morning while I went for a walk.

As I rounded a six-foot stone wall bordering my neighbor's house, I came face-to-face with another of my clients. Tyler was a methamphetamine dealer and a few days earlier had graphically described to me how he and his wife manufactured and dealt crystal meth out of their home. They were clean now, but the thought of a meth dealer living 5 houses away unnerved the hell out of me. Keep in mind that I live in a small suburban town, a classic bedroom community with low crime rates, good schools and more churches than bars.

When I think about it now, my living near this dealer probably unnerved him more than it did me. I rarely saw him again and he and his wife soon moved away. But it put something into perspective. We all tend to see the "drug dealer" from our own viewpoint – usually as someone who is quite different from us. This couple were both professionals, one in education, the other in medicine. They were well spoken and well dressed. Neither had an arrest record and appeared to all the world as a perfect addition to our community – or perhaps yours. It is because of people like this, after a lot of thought, that I chose to remain in the treatment field. I realized that treatment needs people who are not intimidated by drug users and can find rewards working with the most difficult clients.

***

As a medical problem, methamphetamines, cocaine and similar forms of "speed" are a nightmare to just about all who use them (or treat those who use them). Powerful nervous system stimulants, in seconds they cause an immediate increase in heartbeat, respiration, body temperature and blood pressure. This rapid-fire stimulation leads to the sudden death of many from cardiac arrest, seizures, stroke and respiratory failure. Put into a different perspective, these drugs are more than just a problem for individual addicts. They have become a societal problem, decimating neighborhoods and wiping out large numbers of an entire inner-city generation. Having seen the damage first hand, I shudder when I hear "experts" propose blanket legalization for all drug use, letting people make their own choices of whether to use or not. With cocaine, methamphetamines, and other powerful drugs like fentanyl, as seen with so many people, there is little choice. Finally, it must be remembered by those who want to, "let people make their own choices" that the average age for first time drug use is the early teens. Putting cocaine, methamphetamines and equally dangerous drugs in the hands of those whose brains are not fully developed is like handing each adolescent a hand grenade and telling them it is okay to play catch with it, just don't pull the pin.

CRUDE BUT EFFECTIVE

In the evolution of drug treatment, the second change (after the introduction of "smokable" drugs like crack cocaine and methamphetamines) came with a dramatic increase in the potency and availability of an old and well-known drug – heroin. Heroin (def.) is an opiate alkaloid with no acceptable medical use, making it a Schedule I drug – it has a high potential for addiction. Those addicted to heroin are addicted to all other opioids, notably oral pain medications like Codeine, Percocet, Oxycontin and fentanyl. Most addicts begin their opioid addiction after an injury or surgery resulted in the use of pain medication over a lengthy time frame. Injury and pain are also common triggers for relapse when pain management is required. *Recovering addicts need to address pain with alternatives to opioids and close monitoring of all addictive substances. (NOTE: an **opiate** medication is derived from the opium poppy. **Opioid** medication is any narcotic drug, natural or synthetic, that has opium-like effects but is not necessarily derived from the poppy.)*

Heroin, like all opioids, produces *analgesia, (def.) meaning it reduces pain – by acting upon the central nervous system.* It alters the patient's perception of stimuli to the senses and produces a rapid increase in *tolerance*, *(def.)* *a phenomenon in which the user needs increasing amounts of a substance to produce a desired effect.* It causes physical dependence, respiratory depression, gastrointestinal spasms and powerful euphoria. When the Civil War came to an end in 1865, there were thousands of soldiers with painful, debilitating injuries that could be treated with little other than morphine. As a result, morphine addiction came to be known as "the soldier's disease" with countless thousands seeking help for both pain and addiction. Heroin was developed in 1898 for use in treating morphine addiction, the belief being that it was less addictive than morphine. It is not. Heroin is more powerful than morphine, acts faster and is just as addictive, if not more so.

Sudden cessation of heroin use, often after using it only a few times, produces *acute abstinence syndrome, (def.) better known as* **withdrawal.** Heroin withdrawal is characterized by anxiety, restlessness, irritability and craving for another dose. Within a few hours after last use, symptoms of tearing eyes, runny nose, heavy perspiration, yawning and sleepiness occur. Upon waking, more significant withdrawal symptoms occur including vomiting, achiness in the joints and bones, diarrhea, painful abdominal cramps, convulsions (seizures) and cardiac symptoms including weakness, shortness of breath and chest pain. Withdrawal symptoms peak at three to five days of abstinence and last for approximately fourteen days. Longer, *post acute withdrawal* symptoms such as depression, anhedonia and insomnia can last for months after last use, and can easily lead to a relapse.

Heroin addicts often have three options to support their habit – deal, steal or prostitute. Most will deal small amounts of heroin to other users making enough money, at least for a while, to support their own habit. Heroin addicts are also thieves. It is estimated that a heroin addict will commit between three hundred and five hundred felonies per year to support a habit. Shoplifting or "boosting" is the easiest and least dangerous crime for most. It usually takes multiple convictions before facing the chance of incarceration and, since the court usually views shoplifting as a non-violent crime, jail time tends to be brief. Many addicts travel a wide geographic area, often with a partner, to avoid being caught. An experienced shoplifter can support a large habit with very little risk of incarceration.

Addicts find other ways to steal also. I used to see a lot of workplace injuries that provided incredible opportunities for creative addicts to milk the system. While at the HMO, a brief survey of my clients showed that of forty-one heroin users on my caseload, thirty-seven had been or were currently on workers compensation for a workplace injury. Many of these were blatantly false, and occasionally a client would brag openly about scamming the system.

Finally, there is prostitution. Even among addicts it tends to be looked down upon. Calling it the "oldest profession," making light of it or movie depictions of prostitutes as "cool, beautiful working girls" does not do justice to this dangerous, disease-ridden and tragic way of life.

Debbie was a prostitute. A long-time heroin addict, she had a lengthy track record of criminal activity and subsequent incarceration. It is a familiar story if you are working with addicts. One day, during one of our counseling sessions, the subject of withdrawal came up and it occurred to Debbie that I probably did not really know how bad it is. Her description remains tattooed in my memory.

"You start thinking about getting high before your eyes are open, 4:00, 5:00 A.M. You know you're going to be sick so your mind starts working out what you're gonna have to do to get the money and get a bag (of heroin). If you're smart, you saved a bag from the night before, so you won't be so sick. Mostly you don't though 'cause if it's there, you use it all. I'm a real pig junkie, I've never been able to save any." She laughed as she said this. She often talked about needing a "wake up," a bag of heroin just to get out of bed without being too sick.

"You feel cold – you always feel cold when you're dope sick. And it can be twenty degrees outside but you're so sick that in spite of how cold it is you put on a short skirt, hike it up around your ass, put on your coat and go out to hustle. Sometime the only warm thing is your goddamn cigarette. You stand on the street to stare down guys driving by. You want them to stop; you need someone to stop before a (police) cruiser comes up the street and you gotta go back inside. Finally, you hop into the front seat with some sour-smelling bastard who's been working all night and stinks like piss. You give him a blow job for the price of a bag of dope. So you can feel better.

Do you have any idea how bad dope sickness is when you hafta do that just to feel better?"

Tragically, Debbie was murdered. Found dead and stuffed into a dumpster behind a bar. Her murder has never been solved. After her body was found, the topic of risk came up in group. Even I was surprised when all six women in my group told horrible, frightening stories of being robbed, beaten, raped and mutilated by "johns" while trying to earn the price of a bag of dope. The price is always too high – unless you have a dope habit.

When I first started treating heroin addicts in the late 1970's, the strength of dope on the streets of Worcester, as in most New England cities was about 8-10 %. The rest of the dope was usually made up of *cut* which might be anything from powdered milk to baby laxative to crushed medications. An average heroin habit was seven to eight bags per day, occasionally reaching as much as a *bundle* or ten bags. It sold on the street for about $25.00 per bag or $200.00 per bundle (10 bags). We usually treated long-time addicts who had been using for five years or more and all were using it intravenously.

In the mid 1980's the strength of heroin began to increase rapidly along with its availability, while the price went way down. It got as strong as 70-80% purity and was selling for under $10.00 per bag and less than $100.00 per bundle. The combination of lower prices with greater strength and availability meant that heroin addicts now used more and developed much greater habits much faster. The higher strength also created an increased possibility of overdosing. By the mid 1990's at least half were using it intranasally, or "snorting" heroin, under the mistaken belief that it is less addictive and, if you snort it, you cannot overdose.

At this time, many long-term heroin addicts were complaining that the dope on the streets was "weak...watered down...has too much cut in it." It was not the heroin getting weaker though. *It was the addict's **tolerance** getting stronger. The stronger the dope, the more they need to use because strong dope builds tolerance quickly and the addict needs to use more and more to get the same effect. The more they use, the higher their tolerance for the opioid and the less euphoria they feel. This makes them believe that the heroin they are using is weak.*

This is one of the factors leading to more overdoses. Clients get clean for short periods of time via detox or jail. This quickly decreases their tolerance. Then they return to using the same amounts of heroin and subsequently overdose. This occurs because they've lost their tolerance in the period of time they were drug-free after a detox or incarceration.

Another major factor leading to the increase in overdoses is the change in "cut," *(def.) the substance used to extend the amount of the drug.* Most cut was comprised of over-the-counter medications, powdered milk, baby laxatives or something that might add a slight rush to the drug user's experience. Then, by the mid-1990's, drug users found that fentanyl citrate, *(def.) a synthetic opioid analgesic used for chronic pain management,* could be used as a cut. This greatly extended the heroin dosage while making the opioid more powerful. I became aware of this when one morning my first patient reported grinding up fentanyl pain patches and mixing them with heroin. He died of an overdose minutes after leaving my office.

Fentanyl has led to a rapid increase in overdose deaths and is currently involved in 75-80% of overdoses. *Fentanyl is 30-40 X more potent than heroin and 100X more potent than morphine. It is not dispensed in milligrams, (a milligram is 1/1000 of a gram.) Fentanyl is dispensed in micrograms (a microgram is 1/1000 of a milligram, or one millionth of a gram.) It is primarily dispensed through patches, sprays or pills and is used for chronic, debilitating pain, often post-surgery. Illicit fentanyl is notably dangerous. (Random testing recently found that 42% of fentanyl pills contain at least 2% fentanyl, which is lethal for most users.) Drug dealers have no Quality Control Department and since the drug is so lethal, even in miniscule amounts, it is very easy to ingest a potentially fatal amount. This is why fentanyl puts users at extremely high risk for overdosing.* It is tragic to hear about young people who died in their first or second experimentation with drugs that have been spiked with fentanyl. They do not get a second chance at life. (Put another way, a kilogram of fentanyl could kill up to ½ million people.)

Finally, with the increased availability of opioids came expansion of the *drug culture.* When we examine the history of heroin addiction, we see that before World War II, it was usually found in large cities and among the poor, and with certain edgy occupations, like musicians. By the 1950's, times were good and drug habits were not expanding much. Then came the 1960's and drug use began to increase, spreading to the young and affluent. The Vietnam War drove demand and with increased demand came more availability. By the 1980's opioid dependence had crossed racial and economic lines and heroin use was expanding beyond the inner city. Since the mid-1990's, with demands for opioid pain medications continually rising, heroin and other related drugs are found virtually everywhere. It can be said that every city and town has a street, neighborhood or house where lethal drugs are readily available. Oh yes, it is cheaper now, a lot cheaper, and this has effectively created a culture where dangerous drugs are available to everyone, everywhere.

SOMEONE YOU CAN DEPEND ON

Marjorie was the single mother of a seven-year-old son, Brian. A chubby, outspoken girl who made a good living as a waitress, she did not fit the stereotype of an emaciated, depressed and sickly junkie. She was a *chipper, (def.) one who uses heroin on an occasional basis* when partying with friends. Like most, she managed to avoid regular use – at least for a while. Chippers tend to think they are different. They "won't get hooked," and often tell me they can handle it. "It won't happen to me. I only use it once in a while."

Marjorie always said she was afraid of needles, so she snorted heroin. One morning, while Brian was at school, two friends, a couple of whom Marjorie would later say, "I thought I could depend on them…" came to her apartment to share some heroin. Actually, Marjorie had a paycheck, so they came to share that, selling her the dope they would all use together. Marjorie snorted a bag. She said later that she knew she was "going out," but could not do anything about it. Marjorie passed out in a classic heroin overdose.

Her friends were indeed people she could depend on. Rather than call 911, they rifled through her apartment and left. The woman later told Marjorie they thought she was dead, so why call for help and get in trouble with the police. Heroin addicts can indeed be depended on for that kind of thinking. Later, Brian came home from school to find his mother near death on the living room floor, lying in vomit. He will remain scarred by that for the rest of his life.

Marjorie was hospitalized for three weeks and returned to my office six weeks after her overdose. She looked healthy, a little thinner, but was much different. She said, "My coffee table is covered with little yellow sticky notes to remind me of things. I can't remember anything. I can remember up to that day, but I can't remember what the hell I'm doing from one minute to the next." Brain damage. It will plague Marjorie for as long as she lives.

When I last saw Marjorie, her son Brian was waking up in the night screaming. He was afraid to go to school and more fearful of coming home. He was afraid of finding his mother dead. Later, like all children, he expressed his fear in the only way children can, with anger. He lashed out at Marjorie, his teachers and other children for Marjorie's wrongs and his own terrors. Marjorie's parents no longer talk to her and no one, not her son, her ex-boyfriend, her friends nor her employer will ever completely trust her.

Marjorie remained clean and moved out of Worcester. Her memory improved over time and she is again working. The real victim is Brian, who never resolved his fears. He can neither understand his mother's illness nor forgive her for it. He lives in another state now with his biological father.

Marjorie became a victim of heroin that over the years became stronger and cheaper, especially when cut with Fentanyl. As explained previously, the increased strength and purity, as well as the addition of the powerful drug Fentanyl, made heroin more lethal and addictive, with many seeking treatment after only a few months of use. The low price and availability make it possible for addictions to become worse than was thought possible. Tolerance increases with every bag. As a result, the more you use, the more you need. Heroin addicts eventually use almost continuously just to keep the sickness of withdrawal away. It is this simple: the more dope available, the more the addict uses until either the supply, the money or the life runs out.

Finally, a few words on errors and false assumptions about opioids:

1. *Opioids work for chronic pain.* This is untrue. There is little evidence that they work well for chronic pain due to the increased potential for addiction from higher drug tolerance combined with loss of pain tolerance. The exception to this is patients with terminal illness, where the issue of addiction is less important. Initially dispensed for cancer patients, *extended-release* versions of opioids became available to anyone with chronic pain. This increased the risk of addiction, loss of pain tolerance and multiple side effects from confusion to constipation. *If used for chronic pain, opioids must be closely monitored to ensure alcohol and other medications are not mixed in and that the patient's tolerance is not changing.*

2. Opioids *are not addictive if used for pain relief:* This is untrue. At least 25% of those who use pain medications become addicted. Work for a while in any drug treatment facility and you soon realize that many, if not most, started their addiction using opioids for pain. In 2017, 70,000 Americans died from opioids. Since 2020, it is over 110,000, most of whom started with a prescription for pain medications.

3. *Extended-release versions of opioids are safer.* This too, is untrue. Extended-release versions stay in the body longer. Also, the physician should emphasize – no sleep meds, alcohol or other sedatives should ever be used while on an opioid and follow-up by the physician should be frequent. The MD needs to track prescriptions closely to ensure meds are not being mixed or purchased in multiple places.

Summary:

No one makes a conscious decision to become an addict. The younger a person starts, the more an addiction is likely to develop. The medical profession has shown a poor understanding of addiction and its causes with many well-intentioned physicians over-prescribing highly addictive medications.

Cross addiction, (those addicted to one drug are addicted to others of the same family), and synergism, (the combined effects of more than one drug are more than the same amount of either take separately) can lead to overdose, addiction and death.

Cocaine and methamphetamines produce a rapid onset of addiction characterized by binge use. Cocaine has a half-life of one hour, methamphetamines have a half-life of 12 hours, meaning that methamphetamines stay in the body much longer. Both are neurotoxins and lead to brain damage (organic brain syndrome), cardiac issues, mental health problems and violent behavior. Both drugs affect the hypothalamus, a small organ at the base of the brain, leading to problems with heartbeat, breathing, and sexual dysfunction among other issues.

Withdrawal from alcohol causes acute illness, agitation, depression and excess fatigue. It can be fatal. Opioid withdrawal causes nausea, cramping, gastric complaints for 5 – 7 days with acute symptoms of sleep deprivation, leg spasms, insomnia, depression, emotional pain and agitation lasting for two to three weeks. Not usually fatal, opioid withdrawal is severely uncomfortable and craving can last for months. Rapid loss of tolerance after an opioid detox leads to overdoses when the opioid user returns to using a high amount after losing his previous tolerance after a detox.

Amphetamines and cocaine re-write withdrawal. At first there are few physical symptoms. At about 3-5 days away from the drug, there is a pre-occupation with using – this comes just in time for the weekend for many users, so actual withdrawal is not recognized by most. About 12% become suicidal at some point. With regular users, cardiac problems are seen as are loss of sexual function and anhedonia.

Triggers for drug relapse are defined as substances, objects or agents that stimulate drug use. The three most prominent triggers for cocaine and methamphetamine users (as with many other illicit drugs) are: (1) alcohol use, (2) money, (3) people. Methamphetamine and crack cocaine users exhibit few withdrawal symptoms but have a powerful urge to use once triggered.

Heroin, an opiate, is an analgesic (pain reducer). Since the late 1980s, there is an increase in the potency and availability of opioids. Opioids produce a rapid increase in tolerance, causing more of the drug to be needed to produce the desired effect. Addicts experience less euphoria as they need increasing amounts of the drug. Cessation produces withdrawal with extreme discomfort, both physical and psychic. Heroin addicts usually deal drugs, steal or prostitute. This puts them at high risk for death, injury and incarceration. Heroin causes overdoses even when snorted.

"Cut" is the term used for a substance mixed with a drug to extend the amount to be sold. Often used as a cut, fentanyl (citrate) is a synthetic opioid used for debilitating pain and is usually prescribed in patches, lozenges and sprays. It is 100X more potent than morphine. When used as a "cut" fentanyl has been found to be a factor in up to 90% of overdose deaths. Fentanyl is far more dangerous than heroin. A kilo (2.2 lbs.) of fentanyl could kill ½ million users.

SECTION III

THE MAKING OF AN ADDICT

CHAPTER 5
FAMILY, CIRCUMSTANCES AND GENETICS

No one makes a conscious choice to become addicted to drugs any more than they choose to come down with cancer. However, there are personality characteristics and environmental factors as well as behavioral and family traits found in addicts that are not found as frequently in other people. These factors often eliminate much of the role choice plays in the development of addiction. **Keep in mind that these are generalities, for there is no such thing as an "addict personality." No one, single thing is common to all people with addictions.** *Each person addicted to drugs is an individual molded by their parents, experiences, circumstances and genetics as well as by their drug of choice.*

Many of those addicted to drugs live on the fringe of society even before they start using. There is often a history of escalating anti-social behaviors like truancy, vandalism, shoplifting and bullying that start in early adolescence, sometimes in those as young as pre-teens. It is not uncommon to find those entering treatment to have spent early years in residential programs or foster homes. In school, addicts tend to be intelligent under-achievers who lack goals and self-discipline and seek excitement in illegal behaviors.

Frequently, addicts come from families that, whether they are intact or not, lack moral direction. There are often few religious or socially acceptable values to draw upon and a lack of conventional morality, with parents who are dishonest, excessively controlling, have a history of incarceration or anti-social behavior or are themselves addicted. *Many addicts come from families where drug use and excessive drinking are viewed as recreational activities.* Also, poverty is an ever-present factor in many of these families.

Finally, there is a high frequency of abuse and neglect found in families of addicts. It has been said that many addicts grow up in a war zone. It is unusual to meet one who can consistently relate pleasant memories of growing up. They often describe painful incidents of beatings, neglect, verbal abuse and ridicule. Many, when asked about childhood memories, make jokes about incidents of trauma or remember little.

A study of residential drug treatment from the 1970's found that 80% of women in these programs had been victims of sexual abuse. *This may seem high, but it is one of the most pervasive problems that those providing drug treatment need to address.* It is difficult to find accurate research regarding childhood sexual abuse of male addicts, but a substantial number of my own clients, male and female, were abused sexually.

IMPAIRED PERSONALITIES

A high percentage of my addicted clients were a product of abuse: physical, mental, emotional or sexual abuse. Abuse and neglect are among the factors that create a group of mental health disorders called **personality disorders.** A personality disorder is *(def.) a pattern of thoughts and behaviors that deviates markedly from the expectations of the individual's culture.*

There is a large segment of mental health professionals who maintain all who suffer from addictions also suffer from personality disorders. This is arguable. However, there is little disagreement that addicts suffer from personality disorders at a higher-than average rate, one that parallels the rates of abuse, neglect and emotional trauma they are found to have endured in the most formative years of their lives. The Diagnostic and Statistical Manual of Mental Disorders (DSM-5), the primary guide for diagnosing mental health problems, describes those with personality disorders as *exhibiting enduring and inflexible patterns of behavior that begin in adolescence or young adulthood.*

The DSM-5 identifies three clusters of personality disorders based upon descriptive similarities. Cluster A includes paranoid, schizoid and schizotypal personality disorders. *Cluster B includes the antisocial, borderline, histrionic and narcissistic personality disorders. (Those found in the B cluster group are most frequently found with drug and/or alcohol addictions.)* Those in Cluster C include the avoidant, dependent and obsessive-compulsive personality disorders.

Addicts can suffer from any of the ten personality disorders but the four in cluster B are most prominently found with addictions. It must be emphasized however that this is not a fact carved in stone. ***Addictions can be found with all personality types. Factors other than psychological and emotional, such as physical, family, cultural, genetic, age at first use, type of drug used, influence of others and a multitude of additional factors feed into the development of addictions.***

***

The first and perhaps the most common of the personality disorders found among addicts is the ***Antisocial Personality Disorder* (301.7)**.

Mark began life as a troubled child. He was running away from home at age ten because he hated his stepfather. He became a problem in school, stealing, fighting and even getting expelled for setting a fire in one of his classrooms. Mark was born to a mother who had just turned fifteen. She worked hard and put herself through college by the time she was twenty-five. That is where she met Mark's stepfather. Mark never liked this man who demanded all his mother's attention and, when Mark acted out, "ruled with a firm hand." His mother did not recognize the problem for she thought the rigid discipline from Mark's new father was going to help. When Mark rebelled even more, she sought help through Juvenile Court. She would later tell me that this was the worse decision of her life. For Mark, at age 12, was sent to a Boys Home where he stayed until he was sixteen. There, Mark became an accomplished criminal.

I first met Mark in the methadone program. He had been transferred to me from another clinician who warned me to be very careful not to leave anything around that could be stolen. He was viewed as problematic even by the standards of the methadone clinic that handled every sociopath in the city. Mark was barred from the local mall for shoplifting. He stole compulsively, not only to support his drug use, but because he found it exciting. Mark was diagnosed with an **antisocial personality disorder.** *Those suffering from this* *disorder are often referred to as psychopaths or sociopaths. Their behavior is characterized by extreme impulsivity with little thought for the consequences of their actions.* Their impulsivity makes a commitment to recovery from addiction very difficult. They lie and use people for personal gains such as money, sex or power. They often have a history of multiple sexual partners and tend to be terrible parents, neglecting their children. Most notably, judged by their behavior, they appear to have no conscience. Remorse only comes from being caught and apologies and amends are superficial.

There is a high prevalence of **antisocial personality disorder** among those addicted to street drugs like heroin. One of my group clients pointed out the differences between himself, an alcoholic, and the heroin addicts in treatment with him. "Most alcoholics are working, family people, at least to start with. They are usually honest and feel guilty about their past actions. They (heroin addicts) are different. They go bad real young…most were criminals as kids. They don't care…they don't seem to have a conscience. You can be a nice guy and be a drunk, but you cannot be a nice guy and be a junkie."

Mark is a textbook case study of **antisocial personality disorder.** A local department store filed a civil suit against Mark for theft. This was unheard of, and Mark was quite proud of that. They caught him walking out of the store with a basket full of expensive clothes. Since they saw him in the store all the time, they reviewed their security tapes and, by their own estimates, he had stolen about $60,000 worth of goods in a four-month period. Mark was truly a walking crime wave.

Mark was small, of slight build and could almost be described as pretty. In the Boys school, the weak were preyed upon not only by the usual bullies but by staff as well. Mark's stature set him up as a victim from the start. He never could, nor did I expect him to, go into the details of his abuse there. One day he started to describe being tied up in a stairwell, but his words trailed away and he just stopped talking. He never returned to that memory. I did not ask him to, either.

At age 17, Mark was released from the Boys home. He lasted less than a year on the outside before committing an armed robbery that landed him a ten-year sentence. In state prison, Mark continued being abused and re-victimized until, in his own way, Mark learned to make victims of others.

Mark became an expert thief who would target anyone. He could walk out of a store with expensive electronics under his coat and be back that afternoon for more. He once bragged about putting stores in a local mall out of business. His attitude was, "Screw 'em. They got more than I got."

Once, during a period in counseling when Mark's illicit drug use was minimal, he began to talk about having nightmares. He had nightmares a lot and, among his multiple diagnoses was one of chronic sleep disorder. Much like soldiers suffering from PTSD, he regularly awoke in the night screaming and sweating from horrible dreams. Mark said, "I'm always being chased. I'm being chased by ghosts." When I asked about the ghosts, he said, "They are big, they look like fog...and they want to smother me. I can't breathe when they grab me and get on top of me. Then I wake up screaming, and I'm gasping for breath. I'm always screaming." It is not a far stretch to visualize Mark being held down by others, raped and sodomized. The day Mark shared this I made the mistake of pushing him to continue. He suddenly looked very frightened, stood up, excused himself and left. When I saw him later, he had relapsed. He was unable to discuss any of it – his dreams or his fears. *(There is a valuable lesson here for all therapists. Be sure your client is emotionally ready to deal with painful memories before you pursue them, for you can easily trigger a relapse, or with extreme trauma, a psychotic break. Also, remember that sometimes a painful past may simply be best left buried.)*

Mark lived with a girl for a while, a young, badly addicted prostitute. She was physically disabled, homeless and as lonely as Mark. She came from a family with many siblings. Each of them, as well as her parents, were addicts. Most have died or are living with HIV. She grew up being physically and sexually abused by johns and siblings alike and could share little with her counselor or with her support group because she trusted no one. Mark took her to his room, brought her to the clinic, fed and clothed her. He stole for her and hustled for her. They lived together for over a year until Maria got violated and sent back to prison for five years.

Before judging anyone for personal failures, addiction or behaviors that do not live up to my middle-class standards, I think of Mark and Maria. Both, like the previously mentioned "Reynold" did not stand a chance from the moment they were born.

Mark and his girlfriend took in a couple of stray cats and showered them with love. The only time I saw Mark cry was after the police raided his apartment and one of the cats got out. He was out on bail after the raid and searched the streets in vain for his cat. His voice trembled as he told the therapy group how his kitty was lost, alone and frightened, unable to find its way home. No one in the group missed that parallel.

Mark entered the methadone program after being paroled at age 26. He had been out of some type of incarceration only nine months since age 12. Mark is not sure whether he got HIV through IV drug use or from being sexually abused. He said it did not really matter and, in truth, it did not. Sex gave Mark a path to support his habit that was less risky than stealing. He began "cruising" an area of downtown Worcester where homosexual prostitutes earn their money. He never acknowledged doing this although I suspected it right away. His girlfriend knew, but he supported her habit too, so she overlooked it. Prostitution was less risky since he was facing more prison time if he went back to court for another larceny.

Mark came to counseling, like most clients, because he was told to come. In methadone treatment, if you want your medicine, you must come to counseling. If you do not show up, you get thrown off the clinic. Simple. A carrot and stick approach. Mark's treatment is sometime referred to as the "public safety" model, meaning that if you cannot get someone like Mark either drug free or off the streets, you try to minimize the damage he does to others. Keeping Mark on methadone meant that he used less heroin and therefore committed fewer crimes. Mark was never totally free of illicit drugs for longer than a few weeks.

The last time I saw Mark, he was talking about his girlfriend whose parole had just been revoked when she was sentenced for stealing credit cards from "johns," her prostitution clients. He missed her and he missed her cats and was again very lonely. So Mark did what an addict does, he got high. He also got careless. He is back in prison now for robbery and will likely remain there for the rest of his life.

Finally, there are strong indications that heredity may be a factor in **antisocial personality disorder**. This may be so, however, as with the link between addiction and heredity, it begs the "nature vs. nurture" argument. If a child grows up where antisocial behavior is the norm then that is what this child sees as normal. The antisocial personality is often a criminal and there is often a familial history of criminal behavior. There is frequently a substantial history of incarceration, often for assaults and domestic violence. There are three men to one woman found with this disorder.

The psychologist or counselor needs to be cautious, for the antisocial personality often *appears* to be anything but antisocial. He or she is usually intelligent, verbally skilled, convincing and sincere, seeming to want to be your friend and confidante. That is a boundary you do not ever want to cross. They are skilled at using people – and given the opportunity, they will use you.

I recently shared with a police sergeant that I was writing this book about addiction treatment. He asked, "Why do you care about them? They make their own beds. They are all losers and deserve what they get." As I think of Mark and his girlfriend and the many versions of them I have met over the years, I must conclude that they are the unhappiest, loneliest people I ever met. Although Mark is a criminal, a user of others and an extraordinary thief, he began life as an innocent child, becoming one of society's worst nightmares through no fault of his own.

I told the sergeant I wrote the book for law enforcement.

***Narcissistic Personality Disorder* (301.81)** *(def.) is characterized by a pervasive pattern of grandiosity, a need for admiration and a lack of empathy for anyone else's needs. It begins in early adulthood. Those who suffer from this disorder are exploitative, theatrical, attention seeking and braggarts who see themselves as successful and important.* They view themselves as entitled to special treatment. They are easily angered by others who do not meet their needs. Narcissistic personalities see other's problems as unimportant or as weaknesses. They are good at using others for personal gains such as financial or sexual gains and belittle others whom they find threatening, such as doctors or counselors.

In Greek mythology, Narcissus was so vain that the gods forced him to fall in love with his own image. One of my first clients diagnosed with **narcissistic personality disorder** was Jeffrey, a heroin addict. Jeffrey was referred to me by his physician after a diagnosis of syphilis which he claimed to have contracted from his addicted girlfriend. As with most who are narcissistic, Jeffrey saw himself as a victim who was more important to me than I was to him.

On his first visit, I asked Jeffrey a standard introductory question, "Can you tell me a little about yourself?" Most people answer by telling me their occupation or perhaps getting down to the issue at hand, their addiction. Jeffrey's response was, "I'm the type of person upon whom all eyes turn when I enter a room." He went on to tell me how he was working on a Ph.D. when he really had only two years of college. He told me about being involved in his town's politics, a yarn that seemed to grow every time I saw him. I actually thought he might have once been an elected official, after all, he would not be the first criminal elected to office. In reality, he campaigned for his father, who was a small-town politician. When I finally got around to asking Jeffrey about his diagnosis of syphilis, his heroin history and his girlfriend, he criticized his physician's manners, appearance and diagnostic skills. He flew past his heroin history like it was a weekend fling and insisted that his girlfriend was the reason for all his troubles.

Jeffrey, like most with this disorder, made little progress. He immediately wanted to impress me with how together his life was and adroitly deflected any suggestion of change. He rationalized all his behaviors and, when I eventually grew frustrated and confronted him harshly, he left and did not return. This climax occurred after his girlfriend contacted me through another counselor and said she just found out she had syphilis. Jeffrey had been receiving treatment for this for over a month and never told her he had the disease. She believed she caught it from him.

Jeffrey made the rounds of treatment before finally ending up in prison for embezzlement. One of my colleagues read about his arrest and related an incident that happened a few years before when she was counseling Jeffrey. She was driving on Main Street in Worcester when her car was struck broadside. She was not badly hurt but did receive a bruise. As she sat in her car awaiting an ambulance, Jeffrey, whom she had as a client for a few months, barged through the crowd that had gathered and sat down next to her. Without even asking if she was okay, he said, "Marie, I need to talk to you. I'm having a rough day." She said it was the only time in her life she ever screamed at a client.

It is not unusual to find clients with **narcissistic personality disorder** *among the drug dependent population. They are found to have been alternately criticized and indulged in childhood or early adolescence and were led to believe they were "special" with attributes only appreciated by those of high status. They are often physically attractive (Jeffrey was indeed quite handsome) seductive and verbally skilled. They feel entitled to special treatment and use their physical and verbal assets to manipulate others.*

The third personality disorder is the **histrionic (301.50)** or hysterical personality disorder. *They tend to be "showoffs," (def.) constantly seeking attention and are excessively emotional. They are quick with effusive compliments and just as quick to criticize with little reason. Clients with this disorder initially seem to respond positively to praise and compliments but have a continuous need for more. Criticism is viewed as threatening and they can quickly lose their temper.*

In relationships, those with **histrionic personality disorder** tend to manipulate by alternating dependency with seductiveness. They usually dress seductively (this is often a good diagnostic clue) and have problems with emotional intimacy in romance. Close relationships tend to change rapidly due to the need to control others and be the center of attention. It is said of the **histrionic personality disorder**, "They don't make friends, they take hostages."

Sandra was going through a divorce when she was assigned to me. She was on probation for a DUI and was a daily drinker for years, centering a very active social life around local bars. She was quite attractive and one of the primary clues to her diagnosis was that she dressed very seductively – almost exhibitionist with low cut blouses and very short skirts. Normally, I did not like being assigned clients like Sandra because she was pretty, distracting and demanding. One of my supervisors early in my career suggested that I hold a notebook in front of me when talking to clients like this. I could keep the notebook held up high enough so that I did not have to keep averting my eyes from either her breasts or her legs. Good advice.

Sandra cried whenever she talked about Bob, her soon-to-be ex husband. The tears would show up at any convenient time – when she was angry, hurt, lonely or talking about her relationships. Sandra's love for Bob can only be described as "shallow." She met him when they were both married, did her best to keep him from seeing his young son, and blamed his ex- wife for the breakup. She met him in a bar and knew him only a few months when she persuaded him to leave his wife and move in with her.

Sandra saw me in counseling for about 3 months and suddenly disappeared. She met another man who instantly became the love of her life and decided she no longer needed counseling. This man, I later found out, was to become her third husband.

In therapy, histrionic personalities like Sandra are difficult and often non-compliant. They try to impress you rather than address their issues. Female clients with this disorder tend to want male therapists due to the attention-seeking, seductive behavior. They respond to female therapists better however, since they make progress with healthy role models. Males with this disorder do better with male therapists for similar reasons.

Studies of adult children of alcoholics and addicts find a high prevalence of this personality disorder. They are often the ones ignored and overlooked in families that live in crisis. Thus, they learn that creating a crisis is the most effective way to get attention.

The final personality disorder found common to many addicts is the ***Borderline Personality Disorder* (301.83).** One of my colleagues said it best, "A borderline is the client with whom you do your best work. It is the one where you say just the right words. The borderline makes you feel like Freud reincarnated. Your sessions should be training sessions. The only problem is, with a borderline you get to do it all over again, week after week."

A serious borderline is a full caseload. The best diagnostic tool for understanding borderlines is to know all the main characteristics of the other nine personality disorders. A borderline will fit into at least five of them. A client with **borderline personality disorder** frantically demands attention in order to avoid feeling abandoned. *They have a pattern of instability in all relationships (including with their therapist) and often have multiple sexual partners and questions of sexual identity. They view the people in their lives as either saints or demons, depending on their mood and circumstances, resulting in unpredictable reactions to **praise or criticism. They frequently and repeatedly act out with drugs or*** *alcohol, have a high* incidence of eating disorders, suicidal ideation and self-mutilating actions like cutting. They are chronically unhappy and exhibit wide mood swings. They are frequently in bad temper and complain of depression and anxiety. In severe cases, there can be paranoia and dissociative symptoms in which traumatic events or important incidents are repressed and forgotten.

Borderlines, in short, exhibit a whole lot of symptoms. They demand the attention of everyone involved in treating them and make very slow progress. There is evidence that this disorder is genetic, but as with addictions, we once again have the question of nature vs. nurture. *There is also a strong indication that* **borderline personality disorder** *is caused by post traumatic stress disorder resulting from undergoing or witnessing abuse in childhood.* **When taking a history of a borderline, there are often events that meet the criterion for PTSD.** Among these are:

- the client witnessed or experienced events that threatened them physically or emotionally.
- the client responded to these events with intense fear, helplessness or horror.
- they re-experienced the event in thoughts, daydreams, sleep dreams or flashbacks.
- they respond intensely to cues, or triggers that remind them of the events.
- they are avoidant of anything reminding them of the trauma.
- the client complains of an inability to love or feel emotional bonds.
- they have trouble recalling events or important aspects of the trauma.

Why is this important? *A history of these events is found in a high percentage of those seeking treatment for drug dependence. They are the same symptoms exhibited by those who suffer from PTSD due to child abuse.* All treatment professionals need to keep this in mind: the client before you may be difficult, manipulative and non-compliant, but successfully treating this person will require you to look into their history, their families and to the factors that led to the development of their addiction. It will require you to look beyond the challenges of their personality disorders to find the person in need of help.

THE LOST CHILD

Jillian was the youngest of six children. By age 25, she had been married and divorced twice. She was a beautiful, tall, shapely blonde seductive in her behavior. In the time that I worked with her, she lost at least one boyfriend, moved in with a roommate and out after an argument, had a lesbian relationship and became a born-again Christian. I saw her in treatment only three months.

Jillian was the "lost child" in her family. Being the youngest, she was protected by her older siblings from her father, who raped and abused both his sons and daughters during alcohol-fueled rampages. She claimed that she was not sexually abused, but this is certainly doubtful. Jillian at least witnessed terrible abuse. She saw her mother beaten unconscious and witnessed at least one sister being sodomized. She heard the anguish and lived with the terror. At age ten, she was removed by the state's social services, but the damage had been done.

Jillian suffered from **borderline personality disorder**. On her last visit with me, I watched in fascination as she decompensated before my eyes. I was trying to pry carefully into her past, asking about her oldest sister's attempts to protect her from her father. Suddenly, as she talked about her sister, her voice changed, becoming childlike, babyish. She curled her legs up under her and bit her lower lip. She no longer looked at me and began to rock gently in the chair. Jillian talked softly about her siblings by their nicknames and about her "daddy" coming home after a hard day's work.

Jillian was exhibiting **dissociative behavior**, symptomatic of her borderline personality. She learned to escape psychic pain by leaving reality behind. In cases like Jillian's it is often diagnosed as **multiple personality disorder**. I referred Jillian to a female psychiatrist who had more experience with MPD. Five years later she was still working with Jillian, who had made limited progress.

Borderline personality disorder results from childhood abuse. Those diagnosed with this disorder will, in almost every case, have a history of being physically or sexually abused or having been placed in situations of terror, such as being forced to witness abuse of either a parent or sibling. They often carry a concurrent diagnosis of post traumatic stress disorder due to their abuse history and frequently carry another diagnosis of poly-drug dependence related to their poor coping skills.

Borderline personality disorder occurs in six women to every man. It is found in those whose lives are spinning out of control as they fight desperately to control everything and everyone around them. My most long-term borderline client, also my most worrisome, was a male borderline I will call Terry. Our first meeting occurred shortly after I left the hospital clinic for a position with a managed mental health company. His story is a life of pain and abuse. He made progress though, with a simple belief that summarizes my own treatment philosophy. It is called "Moving Forward."

MOVING FORWARD

In 1989, I became the fourth employee of a behavioral health company that provided drug, alcohol and mental health services for Health Maintenance Organizations (HMO's) and other health care providers. The contracts were set up to keep hospitalizations at a minimum, decrease excessive spending and thus increase the profit for the company. Like my previous position, I had my own caseload and was able to see clients as often as I deemed necessary, and as long as management thought it necessary too. The "boss" was the company's owner, who took an approach that some in health care view as sacrilegious. He put patient care before money. "Money doesn't bleed...people do." He told us to treat clients to the best of our ability. This included referrals to inpatient programs when necessary – and we would worry about the cost later. (*This was prior to the widespread use of utilization review policies and procedures which set standards for review of care to justify addiction treatment*.) The boss proved to be an excellent businessman, for the company grew rapidly. But Terry would test this philosophy as well as everyone's patience.

Terry was eighteen when I first met him. Like so many growing up in an abusive home, Terry developed excellent verbal skills early in life. Perhaps this is a defense mechanism culled from the constant need to make excuses and talk one's way out of a beating. This is also why children from abusive homes become such excellent liars, for they learn early in life that the truth quite literally can hurt. Girls found Terry handsome with his deep set, blue eyes. Those eyes were indeed a window to his soul, for they were deep and dark, reflecting the pain and anger of a tormented life.

Terry's parents were married in the 1960's. They were hippies, the generation that brought us free love, counter-culture values and drug use – lots of drug use. It was the drug use that split up his parents, at least that is the reason they gave him. At age six, he and an infant sister were living with his mother. As I worked with Terry over the years, it became apparent that his younger sibling was always treated differently than Terry. Terry looked just like his father, whereas his sister did not. This may have been the root of the terror he endured for years.

When we first met, Terry had been referred by his probation officer after being told to remain clean or face jail time. His offenses were minor, all pot and alcohol issues, but there were a lot of them. He lacked impulse control and saw kindness as weakness. Although he was indeed a victim, Terry also grew into a survivor who was streetwise and could be dangerous. Terry appeared to do well at first, cooperating and providing surface information. Addicts are not good at sharing in-depth feelings, for much of the time they do not recognize them. Until a client is at ease with me, we do a lot of small talk. As he got comfortable, Terry, who had just turned 18, started talking about his girlfriend, a pretty high school junior. The first inkling that something was very wrong with Terry came when he started to talk about "these uncontrollable questions I have to ask her."

Terry had been dating Debbie for about a month. They had barely started dating when Terry became possessive. This was not just a "crush" nor was it simply jealousy. It was a sexualized obsession. Terry became increasingly overwhelmed with thoughts of Debbie having had sex with someone else. Keep in mind that Debbie was a 16-year-old virgin. She had not been sexually active with Terry nor anyone else. Every day Terry would torment Debbie with bizarre questions about a former boyfriend. She had only one previous boyfriend, and that was merely hand-holding in junior high school. Terry would obsess about her having sex and, the more insecure he got, the more bizarre his thoughts became. He would begin by asking questions, repeatedly, until Debbie would cry. Afterwards, he would come and talk to me about it. He would usually start the session by telling me he had "been bad" and asked those questions again.

Typically, Terry would start by asking Debbie about Joey, her former boyfriend. He might ask if she ever kissed him. When she acknowledged that she had, the obsession would quickly escalate into unhealthy territory. "Do you think he went to the bathroom and touched himself and then touched his lips and then you kissed him? What if he was playing with himself and thinking about you and then he touched your lips?" He asked if Joey stared at her breasts, if he ever touched them, if he had ever touched her between her legs. No amount of assurance could make him stop asking these questions. When she refused to answer his questions, he would alternately rage and threaten her, then cry and beg her forgiveness. It is incredible how many ways and with such intensity Terry could ask questions like this. His little high school sweetheart was scared to death. Terry could at once be charming, needy and controlling, so she was afraid to break things off.

One of the most important assets that enables a therapist to provide good treatment is quality supervision. At the behavioral health care company, I was supervised by a psychiatrist who had been in the business forty years and loved teaching. I discussed this case in depth with Dr. M. and grew to understand that Terry's obsession was like a bandage covering a huge, painful wound. His repetitive questions were a way for Terry to avoid facing painful years of physical, sexual and emotional abuse at the hands of the one person he was supposed to trust the most – his mother.

A few weeks into treatment, I noticed that every time I mentioned his mother, even in the most inconsequential way, Terry would immediately avoid responding with a question like, "Do you think Debbie really wanted to touch Joey's penis?" or "Do you think she really wants him to look at her naked?" I discussed this in group supervision and it was apparent to all of us that Terry needed to address his mother's abuse. But doing this meant first stopping him from asking these questions. Finally, what worked was the simple approach – I pointed out to Terry what he was doing and forbade him from asking me any questions until we talked about his mother. It took a lot of work to enforce this, including watching Terry storm out of my office in anger when I refused to answer his questions. Finally, however, Terry realized that he had to do this to recover and began to talk about the relationship with his mother.

When an addict begins to address a history of abuse, especially sexual abuse, he or she will act out. Almost all will relapse. That response speaks volumes about the pain inflicted by sexual abuse. This is why, whenever possible, addicts should have substantial recovery before addressing such a painful issue. If there is not a relapse, then the therapist can expect some type of self-abusing act such as wrist cutting, an overdose or an attack on the person or group trying to help him, which might just be you, the therapist. Terry chose the latter.

Terry trusted me. At least I believe he did as much as someone with a borderline personality can trust anyone. After one session in which he started to discuss his mother, upon leaving the office, he turned and hugged me. He was extremely homophobic. Some of his earliest abuse was homosexual at the hands of one of his mother's boyfriends. He later shared that when he hugged me it was the first time he had ever hugged another man without sexual contact. But as much as he trusted me, the pain of disclosing his mother's abuse left him so vulnerable that he needed to act out. He was too "macho" to attempt suicide, and a drug relapse would put him in jail, so he acted out against me, actually against the behavioral health company. One morning, we found the office had been burglarized. Nothing of any consequence was taken and there was little damage, only minor vandalism. The boss figured right away that it had to be a client, and a little detective work pointed in Terry's direction.

Although there was no proof, only circumstantial evidence, the boss's first reaction was to get rid of Terry and keep him out. It was our psychiatrist/medical director who pointed out that the more someone is out of control, the more he needs to feel in control of something. Terry could only strike out at what he knew. He did not want to hurt me, who was at this point the only person he talked to. He once called me his only true friend, and I provided a safe place for his fears. He did not want to hurt the boss, whom he had gotten to know and respect. He could not yet address the anger at his mother. Debbie finally broke up with him and he could neither hurt himself nor get high. So he acted out by breaking into our office. All that was stolen was toilet paper and some cigarettes left lying around. That itself was a clue. A real thief would have taken something valuable.

The boss, to his credit, (after installing a state-of-the-art burglar alarm) let Terry continue treatment. The boss's rationale, "He's bleeding inside…and maybe we can help him." I am convinced that decision saved Terry's life.

There is a difference between bad parenting and bad parents. Often, parents who love their children simply do not know how to properly parent them. They might unintentionally use their children as pawns in a messy divorce. Or perhaps they abuse their kids by providing bad example. There are those who abuse out of ignorance and those who abuse because this is what they themselves grew up with. There are those who drink or use drugs and do abusive things due to addiction. There are those who do not realize that children are not miniature adults and become abusive when their children fail to meet unrealistic standards. There are those who punish too harshly. There are those who abuse because they are mentally ill. But these people can still love their children and can usually learn to become better parents.

But sometime there are those who abuse their children because they are bad people. These are the ones who abuse children because they can. They have the power to do it. They vent their hatred, pain, anger and spite upon those that are the weakest and the neediest, their own children. More than anything, they abuse their children because they enjoy it. It is not that it makes them happy, but it fulfills an unhealthy need to inflict hurt. Sometimes, they do it just because they can, for it is the ultimate selfishness. They hate their own children. This was Terry's mother.

There was a lot of pain inflicted during Terry's most formative years. As a child of six, he was molested by a babysitter. "I can remember…she was fat and smelled sour, like old sweat. She would lay on top of me and make me do it." When Terry told his mother, she beat him, giving him lumps on his head and bruises so bad he could not go to school. She said nothing to the babysitter and kept hiring her until Terry told his father, who made it stop.

Terry stuttered badly as a child. As an adult, he never stuttered, until talking about his mother. At those times he would stutter so badly as to be almost unintelligible. It was his description of the events surrounding the sexual abuse by the babysitter that first brought this to my attention. Later, Terry's stuttering became a good barometer of how serious an issue was.

There was also a different kind of sexual abuse occurring. Terry described coming home from school finding his mother in bed with a man, whichever boyfriend happened to be in her life at the time. Terry viewed sex as dirty. He obsessively washed his hands and body, especially after having sex, and at times felt nauseous when with a woman. He understood early in therapy the relationship between seeing his mother having sex and his feelings that sex is "dirty." Talking about this led to Terry's first breakthrough. He was telling me about coming home from school finding his mother "humping some pig," when he suddenly voiced real anger toward his mother for the first time. Prior to this, he would only speak of her as, "his mom" and would rationalize her actions and abuse as, "she has problems," or "she's sick." Then one day, while talking about finding her in bed with someone, Terry looked at me and, quite out of the blue said, "That f**kin' bitch. She wouldn't even close the door. I had to look in and see her fat ass getting banged by some pig. She never even closed that f**kin' door and she knew I was there. She knew I could see it…I was just a kid. How did she think I felt?" Terry began crying and wept deeply, looking very sad and then sat quietly for a few moments. He then apologized for his outburst. I assured him it was okay. He was making progress.

Progress is hard to measure, especially with borderlines. I tried to keep my therapeutic goals simple and would ask myself of each client, "Is he or she moving forward?" If the answer was, "Yes," then I was seeing progress. With Terry however, progress was not easily achieved. He relapsed regularly and once became quite violent and was hospitalized for a month. When released, he was on a handful of medications which, addict that he was, he promptly abused. A well-meaning psychiatrist kept him medicated despite increasing evidence that he was abusing his prescriptions. *As with most borderlines, Terry's illness was not some chemical imbalance that could be treated in this manner. It was the direct result of child abuse. But as long as he had medication to fall back on, he could not get better.* About a year into treatment, I was about to give up on Terry and refer him to someone else when he got busted. He was arrested for impersonating a police officer. Like many borderlines, he had a gift for being able to talk his way out of anything. At this time, he had a number of local hookers convinced he was an undercover cop. That worked until he tried to convince the real thing. He was incarcerated for about five months and returned clean and once again motivated.

Terry found safety in my office. He would rage and scream, much to the consternation of the rest of the building, but continued to move forward. After about two years, he began to address the years of childhood abuse. Terry talked about his early school years but never got into details. It seemed he could not remember them very well. (*The inability to remember early childhood trauma is common and the therapist should be cautious not to see this as avoidance by the client when he/she truly cannot recall details of an abusive childhood.*) Terry's parents split when he was about five or six. His father was in jail after a heroin arrest and Terry's mother ran a business from early morning through late afternoon. It occurred to me one day that, other than the one who sexually abused him, Terry never mentioned a babysitter. He was seven, maybe eight with his sister still in diapers.

"I was the sitter. I took care of my kid sister. If she got sick, it was my fault. If she hurt herself, it was my fault." As he talked, his stuttering increased. "I actually thought about killing her...not because I hated her, I loved her. It was to save her from the shit I was going through. I was going to push her in front of a truck...but I didn't have the guts to do it." (It should be noted that over my career I have had three clients who told similar stories of considering killing a sibling due to the abuse at home. Often, children do not get over abuse like this.)

During school, his mother kept the baby in a playpen in the business. After school Terry would take the baby home in a stroller. If school was out, Terry stayed in the house all day, every day. Terry took the baby out once for a walk. It was cold and Terry did not dress her warmly enough to keep his mother happy. When she got home that night, she hit him. Of the incident, he said, "I remember her hitting me with her fist...my head hit the wall. I blacked out. She always used her fists on me."

When Terry was nine or ten, his mother bought a large house with an apartment on the second floor. It was a "bad neighborhood" according to Terry, so his mother decided that he needed to be locked in to keep him from leaving. As Terry talked about this, his stuttering became unbearable.

His mother locked Terry and his sister in a small bedroom with no bathroom. "If either my sister or I had to pee, we had to wait till she came home at noon to let us out. We tried peeing in the corner if we had to go but she would beat us for pissing. Once, I stole an empty can out of the trash to pee in. When she found it she threw it at me...it was all over me. If I cried, I got 'something to cry about.' She used her goddamn fists. She hurt me." This was the only time Terry asked to stop a session. He was shaking, flushed and crying.

I was afraid Terry would relapse at this point. He hung in there however, and we got through the day. On his next visit came a moment of progress. It was one of those rare times when you could *see* the progress. During the visit, Terry started referring to his mother as "Liz" and never again called her "Mother." He was breaking away from her.

Sometime, progress is tangible. The emotional abuse dispensed by a parent like Liz is as harmful as sexual abuse. Terry brought forth another incident, a repressed memory that came four years after he began to address his abuse. With its exposure came a defining moment of his recovery.

Terry was quite young, perhaps six or seven years old. His father had just been incarcerated, one of many such happenings. Terry could not recall what triggered the incident, but it began in his mother's car. She was screaming at him, angry about some childish indiscretion. She drove him to a gravel pit in an isolated section of town. As was her method, she told him he was a "no good little bastard" responsible for ruining her life. This time, she made him get out of the car. "It was late...getting dark. There were shadows and I was crying." His mother locked the car doors and would not let him back in. "I was terrified." His mother threw the car into Drive and circled him, throwing up rocks and dirt all over him, and then sped out of sight. He was left there, crying and alone. "I remember crying…I wanted her to come back. I thought she'd never come back…I'd be there forever. I was afraid a lion or something would come out of the woods and eat me. I didn't know where I was and it was getting dark. I curled up next to a big rock and cried. I was so scared." His mother came back some time later…it had gotten much darker so it was probably at least a half hour. She screamed, "I hope you've learned your lesson…next time I'm going to leave you here for good." Terry could never remember what he did to initiate this incident.

Terry sobbed as he shared this memory. It had come back in bits and pieces over time until he was ready to put it to rest. His tears seemed to purge him. They washed away years of painful treatment and rejection. Terry was silent for quite a while, sniffling and wiping his tears. He finally said, "I have to do something. I have to let them go. Liz is really sick. If I don't let her go, this shit's gonna eat me alive. My father, too. He's useless. He can't take care of himself. I'm ashamed of him. I can't see them anymore. No more. Never again." With that decision Terry broke away from his mother and father.

After he left that day, it occurred to me that this was the first time Terry was able to make a decision about the direction of his life. He was finally gaining the ability to take control of a totally out-of-control world. He finally won a round. He won – they lost.

It was shortly after this disclosure that Terry would sometime stop in just to sit and have a coffee with me. A burden had been lifted. He would bring up the abuse, but it had lost its pain and could no longer hurt him. He acknowledged the horrible treatment he received and said repeatedly that, if he had any, he would never abuse his own children.

Terry consciously cut off contact with both parents, paid off his last "debt" to the court, a probation violation that put him behind bars for a month, and found a place of his own to live. He dropped out of counseling and it would be almost five years before I saw him again. Unfortunately, when clients resurface in a drug treatment program, it is not usually good news. By now I was working at the methadone clinic.

Since I had last seen Terry, he had moved to a neighboring state and gotten into some serious legal trouble. He worked for a lawyer, ostensibly as a runner, a kind of helper/errand boy. He got this job after being defended by the lawyer *pro bono* (for free.) Although he had no money, he worked out an agreement with the attorney to "work off his debt." The arrangement fit Terry's needs perfectly. He got employment, a few dollars, a lawyer to keep him out of jail and excitement. Lots of excitement.

Terry fit the attorney's needs too. Terry was handsome, street smart and well spoken – and would follow orders without question. The attorney liked Terry. He defended him and successfully kept Terry out of jail after Terry tried to outrun the police one night and caused an auto accident that nearly killed a police officer. But there was another reason the attorney liked Terry. The attorney had a cocaine habit.

Terry became a "persuader" a leg breaker who would convince recalcitrant clients to pay their bills. This kept his attorney in money and, with Terry as a bodyguard, out of harm's way. Terry's street contacts eventually introduced them both to bigger and better things – heroin. With this came more financial needs and soon a new angle presented itself. Terry and his lawyer filed a couple of phony insurance claims. These ultimately became his, and his lawyer's undoing. Terry and his lawyer spent about two years fighting the charges. The local district attorney won that war with Terry's lawyer getting disbarred and a year in jail. Terry got two years in jail.

Working with Terry again, I got to see a side of him that had grown. He was no longer the frightened injured child I had seen for years in my office. Terry had by now developed a complex sense of values. His years of abuse and a bad lawyer led to years of drug use. This paved the way first for mental health problems, then for criminal behavior. He could, with little provocation, become violent. But awaiting trial, now over thirty years old, homeless and facing incarceration, Terry found recovery.

Terry was now clean and sober. He began going to A.A. meetings regularly. Personable and sincere, he met a friend who gave him a place to live and some employment day to day. By the time he resurfaced in my office, he had completed a detox and was about to face his final criminal trial.

Terry's family was no longer an issue. He could talk about them as though they were strangers. After years of being abused by his mother, he finally realized she was not worth his time, and he forgave her. *Forgiveness* was the step that let Terry move forward...into recovery and away from his past. His father was now gone, having died from his drug use. Terry forgave him also. Now, Terry could address his other needs.

One of the first things Terry did was ask me for advice. He had been offered a deal by the District Attorney to turn state's evidence against his lawyer. I kept my feelings to myself but secretly hoped he would send his lawyer off to prison. Terry, of course, sensed this and when he made his decision told me I would not like it. He chose not to testify against the lawyer, fully aware that by this decision he would put himself behind bars. Terry said, "He may be an addict, a thief and other things but he helped me, fed me and even gave me a place to live when no one else wanted me. He saved my life. I can't turn on him." Later, Terry saw the humor in this and asked, "Who says there's no honor among thieves?"

There was a final incident that reflected Terry's growth, one in which the word dignity comes to mind. Terry had many hang-ups about women. With his history of abuse, it is no small wonder that he did not become abusive toward women. However, Terry's relationships with women were usually one-sided and often with prostitutes. Then, he met Sally. He met her at a job site where she was briefly his supervisor. Their jobs got terminated the same day the company went out of business, so he asked her out for coffee.

Theirs is no story-book romance. Sally had HIV. She caught it from her ex-husband who was bisexual. She was a beautiful young woman who needed supports in every way imaginable. Somewhere inside Terry was a man with a lot to give. Terry and Sally moved in together, sharing their love and their pain. They fought a lot, never physical, never domestic violence. Terry was not above that, but never laid a hand on her in anger. They described their screaming matches as a difference in philosophy. Sally knew her disease was terminal and, although she denied it, she essentially gave up living. She refused all anti-viral medications and smoked marijuana to give herself an appetite. She refused to see a doctor and would not even tell her parents of the diagnosis.

Terry lived with a different kind of pain as he worked through his past. He tried, and often failed, to live a normal life. In my office, Terry had shaped a personal belief that he must always move forward, his own version of a spiritual recovery. "If I don't move forward, I'll fall backward into my past." Terry wanted desperately for Sally to share this belief with him. By doing so, she would attempt to get better, healthier. He hoped that she would fight her disease, perhaps even beat it. He wanted her to move forward. He begged, pleaded and cajoled. He even brought Sally in to talk with me. The girl I met was a sad, broken young woman, a tired but beautiful girl who had simply given up. She told me that all she had ever wanted from life was to marry and have babies. She had hoped to be a teacher some day. She wanted to have a home and, more than anything else, she wanted to be like her mother, happy and content through the love of her children. HIV took that from her. She felt betrayed and angry at God and at the happiness she saw in others. Sally told me her mother was very ill with cancer so she swore me to secrecy. She would not tell her mother of her own diagnosis to spare her that pain. Life dealt Sally a hand she could not play, so she just gave up.

Most of Sally's last days were spent with Terry. They shared a house in another state until she physically collapsed and moved to a hospice. Terry returned to Massachusetts. He was incarcerated when she died. Perhaps this was best, for he likely would have had a disastrous relapse.

My last message from Terry was just prior to his incarceration. He called to assure me that he would be fine. He said that when he got out, he would have to start living like a man so he could "move forward." He added, "They (his mother and father) aren't in my life now. They were sick but its okay…I've let them go. I need to be a man. I am pushing forty. It's about time." Terry has moved on. His recovery will be a life-long struggle, but he has the support of self-help as well as some good friends. And he has the understanding that he must always move forward.

It should be noted that the biggest factor in Terry's recovery was, and will remain, forgiveness. No one can let go of a painful past, no one can overcome abuse and no one can heal without forgiveness. Terry realized that had he not been able to forgive his parents for their abuse and neglect, the pain would have remained in his heart and poisoned him forever.

Summary:

No one chooses to become an addict. However, there are personality characteristics, environmental factors, behavioral and family traits that are common to most with addictions. Many, especially the users of street drugs like opioids, exhibit antisocial behaviors from childhood. The families of addicts often lack moral direction and there can be few spiritual and socially acceptable values evident. In many of these families, alcohol and drug use are viewed as recreational activities. Also, the presence of abuse and neglect is frequently prevalent, particularly sexual abuse and violence.

Many of those suffering from addiction have personality disorders related to their histories of abuse and neglect. A personality disorder is, (def.) "an enduring pattern of inner experience and behavior that deviates markedly from the expectations of the individual's culture, is pervasive and inflexible, has an onset in adolescence or early adulthood, is stable over time and leads to distress or impairment." Addicts may suffer from any of the ten recognized personality disorders, but there are four that are most prevalent.

*The **Antisocial Personality Disorder**, commonly referred to as the psychopathic or sociopathic personality, is characterized by a seeming lack of conscience, extreme impulsivity, and little thought given to the consequences of their actions. It is commonly found among the users of heavy street drugs like heroin.*

Those with an antisocial personality disorder may appear friendly and cooperative, however they are very good at using people for personal gain. They do not respond well to treatment and need constant redirection to keep them focused. There are three males to one female with this disorder and there is a question of heredity playing a part in its development.

*Those with **Narcissistic Personality Disorder** exhibit a need for attention and admiration, have grandiose behaviors and lack empathy. They often exploit others for sex or financial gain. They are theatrical and see themselves as important, entitled to special treatment and recognition. They dismiss the needs of others and belittle those they see as threats. They grew up thinking they are special. They are frequently seductive and verbally skilled.*

The ***Histrionic or "hysterical" Personality Disorder,*** *is characterized by excessive attention seeking and extreme emotional behavior. They manipulate using dependency and seductiveness. They have difficulty with intimacy in relationships and often dress seductively –which is a good diagnostic clue to this disorder.*

In treatment they are often non-compliant and make poor progress because they fail to work on their issues while trying to impress the therapist. Men make better progress with male therapists and women make better progress with female therapists because they respond to positive role modeling.

*The **Borderline Personality Disorder** is viewed by some therapists as the most difficult to work with. It is said, with little exaggeration, that one serious borderline is a full caseload. They exhibit the characteristics of at least five other personality disorders and frantically demand attention to avoid feeling abandoned. They have a pattern of unstable relationships often with multiple sex partners and questions of sexual identity. They see everyone as either saints or demons. They have unpredictable mood swings and tend to over-react. They frequently act out with drugs and alcohol. They have a high rate of eating disorders, wrist cutting and suicide attempts and are chronically unhappy, complaining of anxiety and depression. In extreme cases, they exhibit paranoia and dissociative symptoms with multiple personality disorder. They are demanding and make little progress.*

***Borderline personality Disorder** appears to be the result of PTSD (Post Traumatic Stress Disorder) from childhood abuse. Their therapeutic history frequently indicates that Borderlines meet the PTSD criteria. These symptoms, found in a high percentage of those who are drug dependent, are often the same symptoms found in those who suffer from child abuse. It is vital that the therapist look deeply at the history of abuse, the families and the factors that led to their addictions.*

Addicts often act out when addressing abuse of any kind and almost all with addictions will relapse when addressing their abuse. Addicts should have substantial recovery before starting to address abuse. The therapist can expect a relapse or a self-abusing act like suicidal ideation, wrist cutting or an attack on those trying to help him/her.

Forgiveness plays a vital role in the recovery from trauma.

CHAPTER 6
THE CLINIC

Managed health care evolved a lot from 1980 through 2000. The Managed care company that employed me made a list of the nation's fastest growing companies twice in three years. The following year, we almost went bankrupt. I had joined the company as the fourth employee and it had soon grown to over fifty. But as quickly as it got good, it went bad. I got out just ahead of a layoff notice. It was 1992 and I now went to work for a large and very busy methadone clinic. It was an inner-city drug treatment program where the rules were simple: you get your methadone each day and go to counseling each week. At that time, it was not even necessary for clients to stay clean.

There are a lot of misconceptions about methadone as well as about other treatments for opioid addiction. But to understand these methods of care, it is first necessary to understand how opioids like heroin, methadone and opioid-based pain medications work in the brain. Opioids, including methadone, are narcotics. They affect mood and behavior and cause drowsiness.

The brain produces its own natural opiates called endorphins. **Endorphins** *(def.) are chains of molecules that act upon the central and peripheral nervous systems to reduce pain and, if over-stimulated by excess amounts of an opioid like heroin or other opioids, produce euphoria similar to morphine.* For example, if you suffer an injury, your brain releases endorphins to receptor sites on specialized neurons (brain cells) and these endorphins reduce the pain. If extra or large amounts of pain medications are added, the nervous system can be over-stimulated and euphoria is created.

When heroin, or any synthetic opioid such as pain medication is used, the brain's receptor sites are flooded with opioids, killing pain *and* producing euphoria.

IMPORTANT: *Addiction develops because this additional flood of opioids causes the creation of new receptor sites on the brain's neurons each time an opioid is used. When the effects of the opioid wear off, the brain's new receptor sites seek more of the drug, causing craving. The brain cannot create enough natural opioids to meet the demands of the new receptor sites, so withdrawal gets worse with each subsequent use.* As more opioid is used, more receptor sites are created, repeating the cycle - with each successive use of an opioid, additional receptor sites are created and the withdrawal becomes a little more severe.

It is this simple: at the start of a heroin addiction, users stay "high" for hours on relatively small amounts of heroin. After repeated use however, the brain needs progressively greater amounts of heroin to meet the withdrawal caused by the brain's new receptor sites. It is common to see addicts using heroin multiple times a day in amounts that would kill a novice user, and they do not even get high, they just fend off withdrawal symptoms.

HOW METHADONE DIFFERS FROM OTHER OPIOIDS

It must first be pointed out that **methadone hydrochloride** is (def.) *a synthetic narcotic, an analgesic (pain killer) with equal potency to morphine but weaker narcotic action, meaning it is effective as morphine at reducing pain but does not produce as much euphoria as morphine.* Methadone's primary purpose is to treat opioid addiction.

Narcotics are analgesics that alter the brain's perception of pain, produce euphoria, mood changes, mental clouding and deep sleep, smooth muscle spasms, decreased peristalsis, emesis and nausea. Narcotics depress respiration and cough among other physical effects. Narcotics such as opioids bind to receptor sites in the central nervous system. They have characteristics of both an *opioid agonist* and an *opioid antagonist*:

First, **methadone** is an *opioid agonist*, (*def.*) *a synthetic opioid that mimics the effects of the brain's natural opioids by interacting* *with the opioid receptor sites in the brain. It prevents cravings and withdrawal from opioids.* This process works in two ways: 1.) Methadone fills in the receptor sites on the neurons that were created by opioid use. This effectively eliminates withdrawal. 2.) Methadone does *not* create additional receptor sites in the brain's neurons like those created by heroin or other opioids. As a result, the person using methadone does not need increasing amounts of the drug to keep from being sick, since there is no withdrawal.

Second, **methadone** *acts as an* **opioid antagonist,** *also called an opioid blocker, that (def.) blocks the euphoric effects of opioids like heroin from the brain. If someone is on an appropriate dose of methadone, they have no opioid withdrawal, there is no euphoria or "high" from the methadone and they cannot get high from other opioids. The key points of methadone effectiveness: there is no euphoria or high and there is little or no withdrawal.*

Methadone, although it is occasionally used to treat chronic pain, (under the labels Dolophine and Methadose) is primarily *administered for the treatment of opioid addiction.* A therapeutic dosage – a dose in which there is no withdrawal for 24 to 48 hours – is determined by the medical staff treating the addict. When the dosage is effective, there are no feelings of sedation, no euphoria and no adverse effects like a reduction in mental capacity or motor skills. Doses of methadone vary greatly with clinics but usually run from 20 to 180 milligrams per day, depending upon the physiology of the client, his/her age, severity of the client's drug habit and additional medical needs such as pregnancy or disease. Initial doses of methadone should fall between 10 and 40 mg. and must be closely monitored for a few days by the medical staff to ensure the patient is neither sedated nor intoxicated. Methadone doses over 180 mg. require close supervision due to possible impairment of motor function and sedation. *A major difficulty with methadone is that it can be hard to regulate the initial maintenance dosage. Too much, the addict will be intoxicated; too little and the addict will exhibit withdrawal symptoms. Since most addicts entering treatment want as much methadone as they can get, it is left up to the medical staff at the designated clinic to determine, through observation and close monitoring of vital signs, how much methadone is necessary.*

Opioid addiction increased dramatically in the 1990's when pharmaceutical companies marketed opioids as safe for chronic pain management. With little oversight, opioid medications were labeled "safe" while neither physicians, pharmaceutical companies nor their distributors could properly define what dosage was indeed safe. *The quantity of opioid administered, the strength of the drug, the length of time the drug is prescribed and the type of opioids used are among the factors determining the safety of an opioid medication for treating pain.* In addition, demand for these addictive drugs spiked throughout the 1990's when pharmaceutical companies not only overstated their safety but also ignored the proven dangers of long-term opioid use. Prescriptions for powerful opioid pain killers like Oxycontin were supplied in quantities of up to a 90-day supply. This created addiction in many who trusted their physician to treat legitimate pain but found themselves with a serious addiction almost overnight. *The number of overdose deaths has quintupled since the late 1990's, with over107,000 deaths per year by 2022. NOTE: **It can take little more than a week of daily use of prescribed opioid medications before physical dependence sets in.** Thus, 90-day supplies proved lethal for many patients who quickly became addicted before their physician's eyes.*

It is estimated that 100 million Americans suffer from chronic pain. Of these, about 10% are taking opioids to address their pain. Four out of five addicts began their addiction with pain medications and at least one million Americans per year become addicted to pain medications. Among Medicare users, (primarily the elderly) 1/3 are prescribed opioids and over 12 million prescriptions are written yearly. There are currently many opioids prescribed for pain relief – and the drugs read like an addict's wish list. *It needs to be noted here that opioids are **not** recommended for chronic, long-term pain until other, less addictive drugs are tried first.* Among the most common opioid pain medications:

Hydrocodone (Vicodin)
Hydromorphone (Dilaudid)
Oxymorphone (Opana)
Oxycodone (Oxycontin and Percocet)
Morphine (Roxanol)
Methadone (Dolophine)
Meperidine (Demerol)
Fentanyl Citrate (Sublimaze)

In the mid-1990's the use of pain medications increased when studies found Americans were suffering needlessly by being denied opioid pain relief. As a result, pharmaceutical companies saw an opportunity to increase sales while meeting a market demand. Add to this the movement to decriminalize drug use and the overprescribing by many in the medical profession, it is no wonder that addiction to opioid medications increased dramatically, killing more and more each year. *In defense of the medical profession however, it must be pointed out that physicians treat pain with medication, not with advice. The problem was with pharmaceutical companies and their distributors who peddled opioid medications as "non-addictive" or "safe" without any proper research to back up those claims.*

There are other medications used to successfully treat opioid addiction. Notable among these is **buprenorphine**, *also known as Suboxone. Like methadone, it is a synthetic opioid.* Buprenorphine's effects are limited and not as effective for heavy or long-term opioid addictions. It has some advantages over methadone, however. Buprenorphine is harder to abuse so patients can take home prescriptions for it. This is unlike methadone which is easy to abuse and is usually administered daily at a clinic site. "Take home" doses of methadone are usually allowed only after the patient has been free of other opioids for at least a few months and is fully compliant with treatment. Buprenorphine users exhibit less withdrawal than those coming off methadone. Finally, the risk of an overdose of buprenorphine is much less than with methadone.

There are disadvantages to buprenorphine however. It is much less effective at reducing withdrawal in patients with long term or large opioid habits. Methadone is far more effective treating those individuals. Even when taken in large doses, there is a limit to the effectiveness of buprenorphine. The financial cost of methadone is low compared to buprenorphine, which can be a massive financial burden to recovering addicts. Finally, methadone is the preferred treatment for pregnant women. A methadone dosage can be gradually adjusted as the pregnancy advances, reducing illicit use and safely keeping them from exposing themselves and their unborn child to other dangerous substances.

Another medication with a successful track record for treating opioid addiction is **vivitrol,** (def.) *an extended-release, injectable dosage of naltrexone. It is administered by monthly injection and does not lead to physical addiction. Vivitrol is administered after a detox and is used to prevent a relapse.* Using vivitrol, the patient must be totally detoxified from opioids for at least a week, otherwise withdrawal symptoms will be immediately triggered. A recent research study indicates that 2/3 of those given vivitrol are clean at six months. **Vivitrol *should never be used if withdrawal symptoms are present or opioid use within the previous week is suspected.*** *(*Prior to publication of this text, a doctor in Australia began implanting naltrexone, providing six-months drug-free for those willing to take it. It too appears to show some success and may be approved for use in America by 2025.)

Vivitrol is also used to treat alcohol dependence, with findings indicating that those using vivitrol post-detox reported fewer days of heavy drinking and better rates of abstinence than those who did not use vivitrol. These results appear tentative as of this time however, and more research needs to be done.

Vivitrol (naltrexone) is an **antagonist drug,** used to block addictive drugs like heroin from activating the brain's receptors. Hence, they are commonly called "opiate blockers." A number of my long-term patients found comfort in the realization that, while using vivitrol, they could no longer get high on heroin. They repeatedly credited this for taking away most of the urges to get high.

Naltrexone and naloxone are pure opiate antagonists that reverse the effects of opioids. **Naloxone**, also called **Narcan**, *(def.) is used solely to reverse opioid overdoses.* **Naltrexone** blocks the effects of opioids and is used to manage opioid dependence. The use of these *opioid antagonists* provides rapid detoxification and can quickly pull narcotic users from an overdose.

Naltrexone is administered orally, and Narcan (naloxone hydrochloride) is usually administered intravenously or nasally. Both block the receptor sites and immediately stop the effects of opioids in the brain. Treatment with Narcan is well known for stabilizing those who are suffering from a heroin overdose and saves many lives each year. Opioid antagonists enable a detox from heroin addiction to take place over a few days or weeks rather than months and sometimes years with a methadone detoxification. However, the major drawback to treating addiction with an opioid antagonist is that it does nothing to address the lifestyle and mental health changes necessary for most to recover from their addiction. There is also a higher risk for overdose, should the patient skip their antagonist and relapse. *It is very important that those receiving treatment for opioid dependence remain in counseling for most, if not the entire duration of their care.*

My son is a police officer in a local town. Prior to this work being published, he saved a heroin overdose victim with Narcan. It took multiple doses of Narcan before the young man finally regained consciousness. He had just gotten out of jail that morning and had lost his tolerance for opioids while incarcerated. My son found his syringe lying beneath him, still "loaded," containing more heroin. He had lost consciousness after shooting less than half the amount in the syringe. Sadly, he again overdosed a week later and died. His heroin had been cut with **fentanyl citrate**, *a synthetic opioid used for pain control post-surgery. It is much more powerful that heroin alone and is today found in about 80% of overdose deaths.*

Among opioid addicts there is strong evidence of **hyperalgesia**, *(def.) an increased sensitivity to pain caused by the use of opioid pain medications.* It is a condition seen in patients treated for either pain or addiction. Pain signals are sent to the brain by *nociceptors, specialized pain receptor cells.* Evidence indicates that nociceptors are damaged by the regular use of opioids causing hyperalgesia. This explains why opioid addicts lose their ability to handle pain and even minor discomfort becomes a powerful trigger for relapse. *This also explains why addicts in treatment exhibit little tolerance for pain and frequently demand more medication. This is not simply "drug seeking behavior." Their brains have lost the ability to handle pain.*

With both methadone treatment and treatment with any of the above-named medications, a change of lifestyle is the primary factor in remaining drug-free once the detox is completed. One of my clients said, "...you need to change the playground, the playmates and the playthings" if you are going to remain clean. Those words of wisdom came from Nick, the thin, chatty son of East European immigrants. His parents barely spoke English but the fear for their only son's life needed no translation the day they brought him to my office.

My first session with Nick consisted of him alternately babbling and nodding off. He was very high from heroin, close to overdosing, and the only way I let him out of my office was in the company of his parents. His mother, who speaks almost no English, cried through the whole hour-long intake process. Nick would later tell me that even after 30 years in the U.S., she was still frightened by what she saw as a strange, hostile culture.

As I finally pushed him out of my office toward his primary physician, I said aloud to myself, "That asshole will never make it." His doctor started him on naltrexone after a week of detox and I figured I would never see Nick again. Sometime I love being wrong. Nick never used heroin after that day and provided a great example of how to make recovery work.

Nick took naltrexone daily for about six months. (This was prior to the production of Vivitrol, which is time-released naltrexone taken once a month.) Taken orally, this opiate antagonist stops the effects of opioids in the brain, making drugs like heroin ineffective. Nick said, "I can't get high on that shit any more, now I can get my life back." After six months, he cut back on his naltrexone dosage gradually until, for three years afterward, he carried only a single tablet in a little tin container for emergencies. During that time, he took it twice after experiencing an urge to use heroin.

Nick's description of the triggers that caused his heroin craving to return is worth noting. Non-addicts tend to think an addiction can be overcome with willpower, especially after a period away from the drug. They ask, "Why don't they just stay away from dope once they're detoxed?" It is not nearly that simple. There are always triggers, either through people, places, things or incidents that can cause an addict's drug craving to return with a vengeance. Remember, the use of a drug – any drug – is the addict's way of coping, relaxing, or handling emotions as well as addressing their fears. Also, the addict's brain has changed. They lost their ability to handle pain and now must develop new coping mechanisms. This is what makes overcoming addiction so difficult. Once the addict stops using, he must develop new ways to cope with life.

His first urge to use came to Nick a few months after his recovery began. He stopped into his uncle's restaurant and was sitting on the toilet in the men's room. This was a place where he used to sit and use heroin occasionally. Bathrooms are favorite places for addicts to get high. There is a seat, running water, privacy and a place to clean your "works," the paraphernalia used to mix, melt and filter heroin. Nick found that sitting on the toilet in that spot triggered a strong urge to use again, so he took his naltrexone and stayed out of the bathroom stall from that time on.

Another urge occurred when one of his old "partners," an addict with whom he had once pulled a rather daring armed robbery, bumped into him at a local store. He looked at Nick and said, "Are you running (using dope)?" Nick said, "No, I'm clean now." Thankfully, his old partner just turned and walked away. Nick told me he felt a powerful urge to get high. He ran to the nearest water fountain and took the naltrexone from its protective tin. (It should be noted that a year later, Nick's old partner was killed committing a robbery near Boston. It was a good teaching lesson for Nick.)

Nick bought his heroin in Worcester's largest public housing project, Great Brook Valley. There are two main roads to reach GBV from Nick's neighborhood, Lincoln and Burncoat Streets. From the day Nick decided to stop using, he avoided those roads. This was no small feat, considering they are two of Worcester's main thoroughfares and Nick had to go a few miles out of his way each day to go to work. There is a lot of wisdom in this simple change, for Nick recognized that, "If I go that way, I'm gonna want to see who's hanging out…just to see if anything is happening. It won't be long before my car will be making a left turn…maybe I'll see an old friend, or someone will want a ride. Next thing you know, I'm sampling the goods again. If I don't drive by there, that ain't ever gonna happen."

Over the next few years, I watched Nick go from a dishwasher in his uncle's diner to a cook, then to a head chef in a rehabilitation program. He bought and gradually remodeled one of Worcester's "three-deckers" a three-family home, got married and has a little girl. He divorced after five years of marriage but remains clean. The most gratifying part of this story, at least for me, is the pride his parents now take in Nick. His mother is not as frightened as she used to be.

THE VIRUS

The most powerful change in the treatment of addictions was due to something no one could have anticipated. It brought about change not only to treatment, but to attitudes. In the early 1980's, those of us providing treatment began seeing a new and frightening illness called GRID, Gay Related Immune Disease. When it first arrived on the scene, it seemed only gay-males were catching it. There was some mention of drug addicts contracting it also, but no one seemed to give it much thought. Nobody seemed to care about "queers and junkies."

By 1985, the disease was now called AIDS, Acquired Immune Deficiency Syndrome. It was seen in gay males, virtually decimating the gay communities in some large cities. And it was now recognized as a problem for addicts, since it was easily spread both by sexual activity and needle use. Today, the disease is called HIV, Human Immunodeficiency Virus. One would have to live on a desert island to not know what it is, what horror it has wrought to the entire world, and how it continues to spread worldwide.

By 1987, the disease was on everyone's mind. In my office, part of our job was to provide some measure of counseling for those newly diagnosed with HIV. Christmas week that year, I had to discuss the diagnosis with two of my clients. Both were recovering intravenous (I.V.) drug users. Darren was a tall, hardworking Hispanic man with a supportive wife. Leo, a small wiry Black professor who was very intellectual and managed to talk his way out of every good position he ever had. I knew them both for about two years and had worked through struggles and relapses until both were now clean over six months. They did not know each other except for perhaps a nodding acquaintance in the waiting room. Neither had children.

Darren came to my office for his scheduled appointment and broke down in tears as soon as my door closed. He had just met with his doctor and had received the news. He had scheduled to meet with me right after seeing his doctor, fearing the diagnosis and aware that he would have to talk about it whether the news was good or bad. Darren sobbed deeply in his grief. He adored his wife and feared he had given her the disease. He talked about never being able to father a child now. He feared his wife would leave him. He was terrified of losing his job because of this and was overwhelmed by the fear of suffering a hideous death. In 1987, HIV was pretty much a death sentence, with the average patient living only about twenty-five months after receiving the diagnosis. (Those diagnosed in 2024 are living at least ten years with many testing negative for the virus after a few years of care.) Drugs to boost the immune system and keep the illness at bay were only in the developmental stages at this time, so Darren's fears were justified – and any words of encouragement were empty.

Darren did what addicts do to handle things they do not know how to handle. He got high. His relapse was brief but vicious and he overdosed, twice nearly dying. He finally told his wife. She was tested (at that time, it took an agonizing two weeks to get the results back) and was negative. Darren put things back together, learned about his disease, began working out and quit smoking. My last contact with Darren was in the mid-1990's. He still had few symptoms and was working closely with a physician monitoring his health and medications.

Leo was a different matter. He was a highly intellectual engineering professor who often arrived wearing a MENSA tee shirt (MENSA is an organization for those with an IQ over genius level). Getting clean was a hard process for Leo, who frequently used his intellect to talk himself into relapsing. This is a common occurrence for intellectuals who convince themselves they are different from everyone else. It is said in self-help programs that no one is too dumb to find recovery, but many are too smart.

Leo's diagnosis also came via his physician. He came for a regularly scheduled appointment and, until he told me at the end of his visit, gave no indication that he had been diagnosed with HIV that morning. Leo's history of relapsing over the smallest problem left me wondering if he would make it through the day. Incredibly, as far as I know, he never used again. However, for me, Leo presented a worse problem. He forbade me from saying anything about his diagnosis. He refused to return to his doctor, refused any medications and refused to inform his wife.

Leo and his wife had a stormy and passionate relationship. They would either be fighting in the waiting room or snuggling like a couple of horny teenagers. I talked to him at length about the need to tell his wife or at least to start using condoms. He refused, downplaying the severity of the illness, using his intellect to talk himself out of doing the right thing. I do not know if Leo ever told his wife. He disappeared from treatment within a few weeks. About two years later, his obituary appeared in the newspaper. He died out of state. There was no mention of family.

That Christmas morning, I sat opening gifts with my wife and children. The death sentence received by my two clients that week weighed on my mind despite my usual ability to leave my job at the office. Their grief and fear put a different perspective on my holiday spirit. I never felt more grateful for my own recovery. Once again, I was given a new perspective on life.

I SAW A TREE TODAY: A LOVE STORY

Elizabeth was a sweet, uncomplicated woman of about forty. She grew up in an immigrant household with a mother who placed little value on education, or on female children for that matter. Her father was a brutal alcoholic who left while she was still in diapers. Elizabeth's mother lacked the ability to survive without a man and her next husband was no better than the first. Elizabeth ran away from home and became a wife and mother herself before her own youth had barely started.

Unlike most addicts, Elizabeth never had to steal or prostitute, always having had a man who loved her and provided for her habit as well as his own. She was probably a poor thief anyway, too timid and shy for the self-confidence it takes to be a good shoplifter. She stayed home, waiting daily for her fix to be delivered by either her husband Danny, or by some acquaintance from that strange community of addicts who sometime take care of each other. When times got tough, like when Danny was in jail, Elizabeth stayed home, locked herself in the bedroom and kicked her withdrawal *cold turkey*, alone like she spent much of her life. Her children, when they were not in state custody, would cook her soup, give her juice or maybe some beer to help her kick the dope. She was not afraid of a detox, she just kicked her habit without medical help because she didn't know places like detoxification units existed. She never heard of methadone until she was sent to the clinic after her diagnosis of HIV.

Like so many, Elizabeth started using heroin when she was young, about sixteen, after the birth of her first child. Her mother had chosen a new husband over her own daughter. Elizabeth never returned home and gravitated from one loser to another until one of them turned her on to dope. At her worst, Elizabeth lost her own two children to the child welfare system. She lived in tenements, cheap rooms and shelters, working menial, empty jobs that fit her lifestyle.

Along the way, Elizabeth met Danny. Danny is a tough little Irishman from South Boston. He looks like a leprechaun with an attitude. A workaholic as well as a heroin addict, he spent days laying carpet and tile or selling used cars, lucrative work and often quick money that supported them both. Incredibly, through 18 years of marriage, periodic homelessness, unemployment and Danny's absences due to jail time, they stayed together. In a strange way, theirs is a love story, for each over the years that I worked with them professed great love for the other. Both told me separately, and with great pride, that they never cheated on the other.

Elizabeth was diagnosed with HIV in the mid 1980's. She and Danny were working together in a skilled trade and had just bought a home. Both had been drug-free and were doing well for the first time. When Elizabeth got her HIV diagnosis, she made the mistake of telling someone where they worked. At that time, fear of HIV was almost as bad as the disease. The company owner found out and "asked" them to leave. They relapsed and never fully recovered. When I met them, Elizabeth was on the methadone clinic and Danny was incarcerated. She got clean and six months later Danny was released and came to the clinic. He remained by her side as she became increasingly sick, loving her until the end.

Elizabeth was uneducated and unsophisticated by most standards. She asked for nothing and took life as it was dealt to her. Hers was a hard life that took her children, her loved ones, her hopes, her dreams and finally her health. There is little time for planning a future when life is lived from crisis to crisis.

Elizabeth came in quite animated one afternoon and said, "I saw a tree today." I asked what she meant and she said, "I was walking here today and near the college there is a huge tree, it must be hundreds of years old. It's the first time in my life I've ever looked at a tree like that." Elizabeth went on to explain, "I've lived in projects all my life in Worcester, Dorchester, other places. All I have ever done was look out my window onto blacktop, parking lots and dirt. I must have looked funny today…I walked around that tree a dozen times seeing how beautiful it is." I suddenly realized Elizabeth was crying. "Why did I have to get AIDS to appreciate things like this…why did I have to be a dope fiend?" Elizabeth cried a soft, silent cry. I don't usually hug clients, but I did that day.

Elizabeth suffered horribly from the virus. She continued to come to the clinic until her last ten days, when she could no longer walk. I visited her bedside to say goodbye and then while she tossed in delirium the day before she died. Danny was with her until the end.

Elizabeth's ashes are probably still at Danny's bedside. He says he will someday scatter them on a hill overlooking the city, but for now they remain with him. He says it makes him feel better knowing she is there when he goes to bed. "I hope I don't sound nuts, but I like to say good night to her." Yeh, theirs is truly a love story.

***

Clients suffering from *"the virus"* as most called it, (until Covid 19 usurped that label) touched me in many ways. There was Paul, both gay and an IV drug user. He was terribly angry until just before he died, striking out at family and friends. Finally, his brother and a local parish priest joined together to meet with him. This calmed him and all were able to say good bye. He died at peace.

There was Pablo. He told me he had the "wasting disease" as HIV is called in some cultures. He saw his mother die from HIV and lost a close friend from it also. Both suffered from severe dementia prior to their deaths and Pablo feared this more than anything. He was a devout Catholic and told me he could not kill himself because he feared he would go to hell. Pablo suffered increased memory loss and confusion. His legs became unsteady as his neurological condition worsened. I had to meet with him in someone else's office because he could no longer climb the stairs to mine. I tried to instill hope, sometime discussing new medications and improved treatment, but we both knew the dementia was getting worse. Pablo died in the same hospice as his mother four years before.

Then there was Peter, who once brought me an ice cream sundae. His HIV was very advanced and, I must admit, because of that I did not want to eat it. Me, who was so proud of not being HIV phobic like so many others. I felt ashamed of myself for feeling that way.

There are many others, some who continue to live, others who have passed on. Some died of "overdoses" which were, in fact, suicides. For me, HIV put a face to the faceless addicts.

SENIOR CITIZENS

Finally, I must address a "specialty population" near and dear to my heart. Mainly because I woke up one day to find I am one. Yes, it is senior citizens, elderly, old timers or whatever else we call older people. We tend to forget about seniors, especially regarding addictions. Young people tend to think that seniors have it all figured out by now and could never fall victim to an addiction. After all, once you retire, your life is either over or you spend the rest of your days doing "retired things," whatever they are. But it does not work that way. Addiction is surprisingly high among senior citizens. There are factors like chronic pain, sleep disorders, changes in health, loneliness and personal losses, all of which feed into the development of an addiction. All senior citizens can become addicted to drugs or alcohol – even those who never before abused substances.

There are factors that lead to the development of addictions that are of particular concern to the elderly. First, those who drank and used drugs regularly throughout their lives but had no issues with them can develop problems once their physical or emotional health begins to be impacted by aging. Aging brings loss of both physical and mental tolerance for drugs, both legal and illicit. *Second,* many develop addictions due to circumstances such as changes in living situation, family losses, difficulty sleeping or health problems. These are factors that often lead to depression. Some of the potential triggers to these problems are:

1. *Retirement*: Most of us define our purpose for living with our employment. "I'm a carpenter... police officer...teacher, whatever." By the time retirement age hits, our entire identity is wrapped up in our work. Then we abruptly stop working. Like the aforementioned "Henry" we can now find ourselves with too much time and a drink or drug becoming our best friend. If accustomed to using alcohol or sleep medications daily, the retiree is a sitting duck for problems with excess free time and loss of identity.

2. *Illness*: It is not only our own health impacted by aging, but the health of spouses, children and friends. I have a picture in my office of three close friends and me taken just before Christmas a few years ago. Eight months later, cancer took one, 15 months after that, death claimed a second one. In the following year, the remaining friend and I were both diagnosed with cancer within two months of each other. I recovered, but my friend became debilitated and died shortly before this book was published. Every time I look at this picture, I realize that getting old ain't easy... because with it comes illness, weakness and loss.

It is after significant losses that many seniors find their doctor too willing to dispense medications, "to help you sleep... take away your anxiety...overcome your depression...help you relax." Also, many fall to the belief that "just one drink" will help them sleep. Those accustomed to using a drug or a drink to help them cope run into problems. Growing older means loss of tolerance for medications and alcohol and, coupled with the personal losses, many senior citizens find themselves alone, popping pills or a drink to cope.

3. *Mental Decline:* It is a touchy subject for seniors, as we all get a little nervous whenever we forget someone's name or where we left our keys. But mental decline is a problem marked by depression, insomnia, memory loss, anxiety and loneliness. For a few years, I delivered meals

at Christmas to senior citizen shut-ins. It is disheartening to find elderly alone at the holidays. Many no longer have spouses or other family members. Time and circumstances have taken friends, and children have moved away with their own young ones. Loneliness leaves many sad, seeking solace in the only way they know – with a drink or medication to lift their spirits. This only feeds into more isolation, depression and mental decline.

4. *Family losses and conflict*: Like mental decline, this too is a touchy subject for seniors. Children are grown and gone away, and even grandchildren, if there at all, build their own lives and families as they enter adulthood. Spouses die or become chronically ill. Worse still, one partner becomes disabled, leaving the other as the primary caretaker. Once again, loneliness becomes an unhappy companion for too many seniors. Ghosts of past mistakes, those that led to divorce or abuse, leave many families scarred and far too many living with regrets that lead to seeking relief through alcohol and drugs.

THE PRICE OF GROWING OLD

In the later years of life, drug use, particularly prescribed tranquilizers, sedatives and pain medications, as well as alcohol become dangerous. When we age and our tolerance diminishes, the effects of these cause rapid damage and the body recovers less quickly. Drugs and alcohol metabolize slower and both brain and body are easily damaged by their effects. The effects of these substances may mimic other mental, social or physical problems such as dementia or depression or even common medical problems such as diabetes. **As a result, there are signs and symptoms of drug and alcohol abuse in seniors** that need to be addressed by a professional *before* medication is used:

1. *Memory Problems*: "Blackouts" (periods of time you cannot recall after you have been drinking or taking medications). These need to be addressed with your physician immediately. This is not a good symptom and can indicate a significant problem with alcohol or drugs. A friend recently told me that her 72-year-old mother calls her every evening repeating things over and over and is slurring her words ever-so-slightly. When confronted, her mother sometimes does not remember making the calls. Her daily glass of wine has become much more over the last few years and is affecting both mood and memory.

2. *Sleep Problems*: Insomnia comes with aging and a change of lifestyle as we work, socialize and exercise less. We often need less sleep. Also, it is not unusual to be troubled by aches and pains from arthritis or other chronic conditions that can interfere with sleep. Be very cautious of any and all "sleep aids," as well as pain medications or regular alcohol use to "help" you sleep. Many of these are highly addictive and lead to trouble. A simple word of advice shared by an elderly friend, "Get used to it…no one dies from lack of sleep."

3. *Mental Health Disorders*: Aging, coupled with physical ills, loss of loved ones, family moving away, boredom and loneliness take a terrible toll on us as we age. Often worsened by strong medications, the impaired systems of senior citizens leave many with sadness and fears that interfere with their lives and terrify their families. Depression and related mental health symptoms can be difficult to treat, since most physicians treat them by adding more medications. In one respect, the very young and senior citizens have this in common – both can be negatively affected by medications far more than mature and healthy adults.

4. *Chronic Pain*: This is the "two-edged sword" facing many senior citizens. Medications used to treat chronic

pain are often addictive, causing a litany of problems, but without them, the pain can neither be tolerated nor treated. *It is vital for senior citizens to seek safe, non-addictive alternatives.* This includes physical therapy, braces and lifts, regular exercise and stretching. Seek alternative approaches to pain from your medical provider whenever possible as alternatives to medications.

5. *Injuries:* This too, comes with the aging process. Falls, skin infections, unexplained bruising and balance issues can indicate loss of coordination, muscle weakness, hygiene issues and even major bleeding problems. Add alcohol or other drugs to the mix and senior citizens become high risk for injuries. Coupled with loss of appetite and changes in sleeping habits, alcohol and drugs leave seniors with a lot of issues that impact weight, body image, mental status and overall physical health.

6. *Isolation:* This problem is seen with many seniors. The life that was once active with work, hobbies, sports and raising a family is now reduced to once-a-week visits from family or an occasional shopping trip. There is a loss of interest in physical and mental activities that feeds into loneliness and grief, particularly among those who live alone or are recently widowed. Too many seniors spend their days staying home, watching TV, avoiding others and sipping a drink or taking a pill to push away the blues. Isolation not only mimics depression but causes it. This feeds into the use of alcohol and pills to feel better, a disaster for seniors finding themselves alone.

Remember, many physical and emotional health problems come with aging but will be made much worse by the use of drugs and alcohol. It is vital to recognize potential problems and to be open and honest with yourself and others if you are having concerns about substance abuse – yours or a loved-one's. Tell your doctor if you have any questions or thoughts about these issues. Never minimize your alcohol or drug use to *anyone*. And remember…no one points something out unless it is there. *If you or someone in your life suspects that you have a problem due to drugs or alcohol, you probably do.*

Summary:

Heroin, methadone and opioid-based pain medications all work similarly in the brain. The brain produces natural opioids called endorphins which reduce pain and, if over-stimulated by additional opioid pain medication, produce euphoria. Opiates are derived from the opium poppy. Opioids is a more generic term referring to both natural and synthetic chemicals that have an analgesic or opium-like effect (pain killing) but are not necessarily derived from the opium poppy.

Addiction is created when drugs like heroin or opioid pain medications flood the brain's opiate receptor sites and create new receptor sites on the neurons (brain cells) with each use. These receptor sites seek more of the drug each time an opioid is used, creating more craving and withdrawal with each use.

Methadone is used primarily for the treatment of opioid addiction. Methadone is a synthetic opioid with characteristics of both an opioid antagonist and an opioid agonist. An opioid antagonist blocks the euphoria of opioids while an opioid agonist reduces craving and withdrawal.

Addiction grew in the 1980's when addictive opioid pain killers such as Oxycontin were prescribed for up to 90 days with little medical monitoring. One week of use is enough to cause physical dependence to begin. Four of five addicts began their addiction with prescribed pain medications. Opioids are not recommended for chronic, long-term pain unless other, less addictive medications are tried first.

Fentanyl (citrate) is a highly addictive pain medication often used post-surgery and is administered in patches, pills and nasal sprays. It was initially touted as non-addictive by drug companies and their distributors but has led to thousands of overdose deaths. Today, it is frequently used as a cut with heroin or other illicit drugs and is directly related to the massive increase in opioid deaths nationwide. It is used alone or mixed with other substances.

In addition to Methadone, medications such as, buprenorphine (suboxone) and vivitrol (naltrexone) as well as others are used to treat opioid addiction. They have advantages and disadvantages over methadone:

Buprenorphine is not as addictive as methadone, but causes less withdrawal and has a lower risk of overdose. Methadone is more effective for long-term and large habits and is much lower in cost, is safer and more effective during pregnancy.

Vivitrol is an opioid antagonist. It blocks the effects of heroin from activating the brain's opioid receptors. It is an extended release, injectable form of naltrexone. Those using it must be detoxified for at least one week. It is usually administered monthly by injection. It does not lead to physical addiction and is used mainly to prevent a relapse. It should never be used if withdrawal is present or if opioids have been used within the previous week.

Naloxone and naltrexone are pure opioid antagonists that reverse the effects of opioids. Naloxone, (Narcan) administered nasally or intravenously is used to reverse overdoses. Naltrexone, taken orally, blocks the effects of opioids and is used to manage opioid dependence. Those in treatment for opioid dependence should remain in counseling in order to change their lifestyle.

In the early 1980's, treatment and attitudes towards addiction changed dramatically with the coming of HIV.

Senior Citizens are a neglected population with little research done into their addictions. Addiction is high among seniors due to chronic pain, sleep disorders, loneliness, losses and changes in physical health. Those who drank or used drugs earlier in life can become affected once their physical or mental health begins to fail. Addiction can develop due to changes in living situations, losses and sleep problems. Potential issues triggering addiction are:

Retirement,
Illness exacerbated by over-medicating,
Mental decline,
Family losses and Conflict

As we age, tranquilizers, sedatives, pain meds and alcohol become increasingly dangerous. Tolerance diminishes, damage occurs easily and the body recovers slowly. Drug problems often mimic dementia, depression or common medical problems like diabetes.

Signs and Symptoms of drug and alcohol abuse in Seniors:
1. *Memory problems (blackouts). There can be many causes of blackouts, but they should be examined as possible causes among drug and alcohol users.*
2. *Sleep disorder*
3. *Mental Health disorders*
4. *Chronic pain*
5. *Injuries*
6. *Isolation*

The use of alcohol and drugs worsens all health symptoms caused by aging.

SECTION VII

RECOVERY –
STARTING A NEW LIFE

CHAPTER 7
RECOVERY AND GROWTH

Recovery from addiction is hard to define. By itself, abstinence from alcohol or drugs is not always viewed as recovery, yet it is a vital part of the process. Abstinence is simply "being dry," as in being free from alcohol. However, i*n recovery programs, most of which follow the Twelve-Step model, the emphasis is on recovery beyond just **physical** abstinence. It extends to recognizing and moving past the unhealthy behaviors that accompanied drug or alcohol use at the start of the addiction. It pursues changes in thinking, behaviors and attitudes by seeking self-improvement.* This makes the process of achieving recovery easier and the results more long-lasting. It also puts the recovering addict in a better position to help others recover.

There are four (4) sections of recovery. The initial part of recovery is often a detoxification, which addresses the **physical** part of an addiction.

(1) **Physical** recovery treats the body and removes the effects of withdrawal but does not address other parts of the addiction. However, changing habits and behaviors can lead to improvements in physical health, which starts the recovery process.

(2) **Mental** recovery comes as rehabilitation programs including medication, counseling and psychotherapy treat the mind and improve mental health. These increase one's understanding of the behaviors related to their addiction. They address triggers for relapse and related mental issues that led to the development of the addiction in the first place.

(3) **Chemical** recovery occurs within the brain affecting neural responses to stressors such as fear, pain, anger, losses and loneliness.

With chemical recovery, the brain develops internal strengths that over time do not require the assistance of a drug to face stressors.

(4) *Value* or *spiritual* *recovery, often the most important part of recovery, is changes and improvements in the value system of the person seeking recovery. It is recognizing, clarifying and attempting to live up to an acceptable set of personal and societal values.* For many, this means a return to or the development of some type of faith, more emphasis on personal responsibility and attempts at self-improvement.

Regardless of how it is defined, *most who recover from addictions develop a recognizable improvement in their value system, either through renewed faith in a "higher power," establishment of new personal standards, or by consciously committing to some sort of moral change in important areas of their life.*

DEBATING THE DEVIL

Perhaps this story will provide an understanding of value or spiritual recovery. For it is the story of a bad man, *bad by his own admission* who, although he remains far less than perfect, has worked daily to undo his past and become someone better.

Barry's burn scars were the worst I have ever seen. Not only was his skin burned off, but the majority of tissue on his arms, legs and torso was burned away to the bone. Five years prior to entering treatment, Barry was doing some plumbing when there was an explosion. It knocked him to the floor and severed an electrical cable. He lay on his back in boiling water while an electrical charge cooked the flesh off his body. He claims he never lost consciousness, but that his soul left his body and he visited the afterlife. Barry did not see any bright lights or heavenly beings, however. Barry went to Hell.

Barry was very convincing. His hands and arms were nearly useless. His fingers were clenched in a permanent partial grip. They were almost totally immobile and had no feeling. Barry demonstrated this by banging his hands against the wall in the group room. The flesh, muscle and fingernails were burned off hands that appeared to be more skeletal than alive. He lifted his shirt to show the group members the scars on his torso and I thought I was going to need my CPR training for a couple of them. His scalp was burned off the back of his head and it was now a mass of skin grafts over a skull. He removed his cap in my office once to show me and I thought I would be the one needing CPR.

Barry was not a nice guy…at least not before the accident. He had two separate families, a large number of kids and never bothered to divorce his first wife before taking up with a second one. He was a tough, barroom-brawling dock worker who drank, used any drug available, worked and played hard. Like so many who lived life through the 1970's and 80's, once introduced to drugs he quickly learned to steal, deal and con in order to survive.

Barry was dismantling a boiler in an inner-city tenement when the explosion occurred. He described the incident in graphic detail during the "newcomers" methadone group on our first night. This was the time when members would customarily introduce themselves. He said he remembered lying on the basement floor, in horrible pain and unable to move as electricity surged through him. He said the water from the boiler was bubbling all around him and he could not breathe. Suddenly, he found himself descending through a "sand-colored tunnel…not a bright light, not a white tunnel like they always describe in those after death experiences…" When he passed through the tunnel, Barry met the Devil. He said that all around the devil were little creatures that resembled people with pig-like heads. They were the devil's helpers. The Devil himself was tall and thin with a bony nose. He was wearing a black cape with gold lining. Everything around him was colorless, gray and brown.

"I was in horrible pain…the worse pain you can ever imagine. The Devil told me that he would take my pain away…I would never have to suffer again if I would give him my soul. I said, 'No' and I kept saying, 'No.' He said I would feel good and the pain would stop. I hurt something unbelievable…but I said, 'No'…I wanted another chance."

"The next thing I knew, the electricity shut off and I could stand up. I stood and walked up about five stairs and out the door where there was a phone. I must have called 911 – or someone did. I remember walking up those stairs and the veins in my arms were hanging off like strings…they were just dangling from my arms, burnt right off me."

Barry was in and out of a coma for over a year. Prior to the accident, he weighted 240 lbs. When he awoke from the coma, he weighed 110 lbs and had to be carried everywhere. It was a month before he could take tentative steps. After sixteen months, Barry was released to return home. There was no home left. His second wife had moved on. His first wife told him he looked hideous and neither she nor the children wanted him back. Although he talked very little about it, Barry believed his appearance was so frightening that his children could not handle it. Barry migrated to Worcester, Massachusetts, disabled, disfigured, alone, lonely and broke. It had been five years since the accident and he had received almost nothing from the insurance companies, the property owners nor the man who had hired him – all while attorneys bounced liability back and forth. When I met Barry, he was living above a convenience store in downtown Worcester. His constant companions were pain and loneliness. "Even the hookers don't want me." I found it unnecessary to ask him why he returned to heroin use. (It must also be noted here that Barry returned to heroin after four years of opiates for his pain were rapidly discontinued.)

When Barry finished telling the group about his injuries, he held up his hands. They looked more like some strange sculpture than hands. He told the group, "I got a second chance. All my life I used these hands for bad things, now I'm going to use them for something good. I'll do something positive with my recovery."

I am unsure how much good Barry ever accomplished, but there certainly were changes. He made amends to his mother and father. They lived in rural Massachusetts near the Berkshire Hills. Simple people, his father was a farmer, his mother a housewife. Barry said he had, "…kicked them to the curb," and never contacted them unless he needed something. Of leaving home at sixteen with multiple arrests and drug abuse issues, Barry said softly, "I embarrassed them…I hurt my mother and she didn't deserve the shit I put her through." Just a few months prior to his mother's death,

Barry made amends and went to live with them, helping his dad with his mother's final care.

I was pleasantly surprised when one day I was summoned to the front desk at the methadone clinic to meet some visitors. Waiting for me was Barry. Out in the car, unable to walk by this time, was his mother with his father at the wheel. Barry wanted to introduce me, "his friend," to his mother and father. His mother was very ill and died within two months. But that morning she grasped my hand and smiled at me and said, "Thank you for helping my Barry. You have answered my prayers." In a business without a lot of thanks, that one made me cry.

Barry had less success making amends to his oldest daughter. She was badly hurt when he left her mother, his first wife. He tried to meet with her but to no avail. She had her own family now and did not want her father in her life nor in the lives of her children. Barry's recovery taught him to understand, though. "I can forgive her for not wanting to see me. I hurt her very badly. I have to accept what I cannot change. I can only ask her forgiveness."

Barry's recovery was indeed *value recovery*. He did not "get religion," he did not start preaching nor reading the Bible. He did not start attending church. He just changed his values for the better, allowing him to understand his daughter's anger, ask her forgiveness and accept her decision. Value recovery enabled Barry to make amends and answer his dying mother's prayers. And it helped him to accept his own disabilities. Perhaps, more importantly, it allowed him to forgive himself. That *is* Value (or Spiritual) Recovery.

As found with so many of my clients, there is a touch of humor in Barry's story. The therapy group with whom Barry shared his journey to Hell was made up of some of the most dangerous people I ever worked with. Four of the ten were paroled "lifers" with murder convictions. One was a professional pickpocket and mugger. Another was a bank robber. All were ex-convicts with histories of violence, including the two women in the group. They were thieves, muggers, prostitutes and gang members. As Barry related his after-death meeting with the Devil to this group of bad guys, I looked at their faces. If nothing else, Barry's story scared the devil out of them for at least that evening. They all looked like they had "found religion." You could read their thoughts... "If this guy's story is true, I'm in deeeep shit..."

***

Discussing evil, like discussing God, religion, faith or spirituality, treads very shaky ground in a book about addiction. There is a risk of injecting morality back into the mix. I do not want to do that and apologize to those who find mention of such topics in a book like this to be offensive. However, Barry's encounter with the devil brings to mind two very unpleasant people – the only two I've ever met whom I felt to be truly *evil*. Neither of them was a client. They were the "loved ones," whose terrible actions gave them joy while causing personal agony to those they purported to love. Evil is a strong word, but it is the only word I have ever found to describe these two.

A BAD MOTHER

Philip was fourteen, referred by juvenile probation for counseling to address a lot of acting out behaviors: shoplifting, vandalism, truancy, drinking, pot use – and a recent suicide attempt. His mother was a tall, attractive professional – and the coldest human being I have ever met. I asked her into my office after Philip's second visit, for it quickly became apparent that something was very wrong with her son. Adolescent boys are not good at describing themselves. They usually tell you a little about their interests and maybe about school. Philip, a tall, slender boy with a soft voice and flat affect began by telling me he was "ugly...my face is too big...I got these scars (from acne), my face is too wide...I'm a freak. I scare others. Even my kid brother is afraid of me." Then he added, "My mother won't touch me...she won't talk to me because I'm so bad."

In subsequent visits I learned that Philip was adopted and knew little about his actual birth parents. His adoptive mother gave birth shortly after Philip arrived and bonded only with her biological child. As time went on, her feelings for Philip, if they were there at all, turned to hatred. Then, maybe because he acted out, perhaps because she feared the consequences of her own treatment of Philip, her hatred reached a truly malevolent level. Upon my first meeting with her, she told me that she wanted Philip to die. She stared into my eyes as though to challenge me and stated, "I don't care if he dies. I wish I'd never adopted him…he ruined my life." I expressed my concerns for his mental health considering his recent suicide attempt. She added, "He's getting more and more crazy…and I don't care. Actually, I'm glad."

I spent an agonizing hour with Philip's mother. She described consciously abandoning Philip to raise himself. There was no guidance, no nurturing. Philip once told me that he wanted more than anything to please his mother. But when he sought attention, she ignored him. Children will get attention one way or another though, and Philip learned that acting out got him screamed at and verbally assaulted. In the loneliness of an abandoned child's mind, this was better than the non-existence of being totally ignored.

When Philip and his mother left that day, I felt relieved that she was out of my office. Not before nor since have I ever felt more uncomfortable by the mere presence of someone. Before me was a woman who went to extra measures to hurt her own child. She took pleasure in it, and openly admitted that she hoped to drive him to suicide. She was doing a good job at this.

I immediately called the referring probation officer. His first words described my own feelings completely. "Did you meet this kid's mother? What a no-good f**king, disgusting piece of shit. She wants to kill her own kid by driving him crazy. (I decided right there that I liked this guy…he speaks my language.) She is the most evil b***h I've ever met." We decided that the only way to save this boy's life was to get him out of the home immediately. Within a week, the P.O. got Philip placed in a local group home for troubled teens where he remained until his eighteenth birthday. I am convinced that he would be dead today were it not for this intervention. The probation officer tells me that Philip, now in his mid-twenties, is active in a support program and has a girlfriend. He works with troubled teens and is pursuing a college degree. He no longer sees his adoptive mother.

I will always be grateful to that probation officer for saving Philip's life.

THE SMILE

Stacia is an East European immigrant. A simple woman, uneducated and naïve, she raised her three children without incident until her husband dropped dead of a sudden heart attack before age 50. Stacia was now almost without income, unskilled, frightened and very lonely. Stacia's world was one of hard working, hard drinking people for whom getting drunk together was the center of most social activities. Stacia described her family and friends sitting around the kitchen table with a bottle of vodka, talking, fighting and even sleeping in their chairs while downing alcohol by the glass for two and three days at a time. Her father was an abusive alcoholic and at least one brother was a heroin addict. (Stacia's brother came to me years before begging for help. He was in terrible withdrawal, physically very ill and vomited in my wastebasket. Of course, he had no medical coverage, so I had to stick my neck out to get him hospitalized. He promptly thanked me by getting arrested walking out of the hospital with a TV under his arm. Further proof that no good deed goes unpunished.)

Stacia and her first husband owned a three-family home within three years of arriving in America. Like many who came from countries where you need to work around-the-clock just to survive, they saved every penny and borrowed from other family members to secure their part of the American Dream. Soon, they brought other family members over who also worked hard while sharing their residence. They began raising their children in the three-decker.

Stacia was referred to me for counseling after an arrest for Driving Under the Influence of Alcohol. Our first few meetings consisted of the usual information gathering and an educational component, much as I did with other DUI referrals. There was a difference, however. Her new husband came along on the second visit. He said he wanted to meet me and learn about addiction, so with Stacia's approval, he sat in on an educational session. Outwardly, Stacia's new husband appeared to be an asset. Left alone with three daughters, little income and barely literate in English, Stacia needed someone who could care for her and her children. She wanted a man who could emotionally and financially support her family and one who would not feed into the chronic alcoholism so evident in her family. She found all this in Benny. Or so it seemed. Benny had other plans.

Benny owned a successful business. He was heavily involved in civic activities, well-liked, smiling and friendly. For that matter, that smile was his most notable feature. Benny was always smiling. That is what I found strange. When I met him, Benny went to great lengths to describe Stacia's alcoholism. He was there when she was arrested and seemed absolutely gleeful describing her arrest, her humiliation and her dependence upon him now for all her needs. One of my colleagues even picked up on it from a brief conversation with him. "Is it my imagination," she asked, "or is he thrilled that his wife is an alcoholic?"

Often, an arrest is a good thing that creates a crisis, forcing an alcoholic or addict to address the addiction. That was not the case with this family. Benny did not care if Stacia stopped drinking. He enjoyed watching her struggle. She cried easily and often, and Benny would chuckle and grin, a toothy, Cheshire cat smile as he watched her struggle in distress. My instincts kicked in. I did not like Benny because I did not trust him. Since he was not my client though, I avoided him and began working with Stacia on a weekly basis. She became less open and quite guarded with her words and disclosures. I assumed this was just part of her recovery process though, since she was now remaining sober.

Upon arriving one morning, I found Stacia and her youngest daughter, a cute two-year- old, (Benny's child) awaiting me. Stacia appeared cold and angry and asked to see me right away. Even my first scheduled appointment sensed something wrong. He simply said, "Go ahead, I'll wait. This looks important."

When I closed my office door, Stacia turned to her daughter and said, "Go ahead, tell Mr. Daley what you told me...you can tell him, it's okay." The little girl was a cute, fair skinned, blonde with ponytails. Her eyes were huge, frightened. Her voice was barely audible, but she graphically described her father's actions.

Stacia had gone to visit a friend for the evening and left their daughter in Benny's care. The other two children went with Stacia but the little girl was not feeling well and Benny offered to watch her. Alone with the child, he gave her a bath and, at some point, perhaps after he felt sufficiently in control, he sodomized her. I felt repulsed as I listened to this beautiful child's words. She described him removing his trousers, "He had a stick in his hand…it was all red…he put it in my mouth. It made me choke." The child sat quietly, emotionless, staring ahead. Not yet three years old, I was unsure as to how much she really understood what had been done to her. Stacia was overwhelmed, but for once she was not crying. "I want to kill him, but I'd go to jail. My kids need one parent anyway."

Per the laws of Massachusetts, I called the local Child Protection office. I also called a child psychologist for the little girl. On advice of our legal department, Stacia left our office and got a "209A", also called a restraining order, keeping Benny away from the family. The following day, Benny's attorney called. He tried to determine whether I, or perhaps Stacia, had "planted" the idea into the child's mind. He pointed out that Stacia was the alcoholic and did his best to discredit mother and child – and me. He assured me that this would end up in court.

About a week later, Stacia disclosed that Benny once raped her at gunpoint in front of her oldest daughter. That daughter would not meet with me, for she left town and subsequently dropped from sight. This girl had been terribly traumatized by the death of her father. Stacia told me that her daughter once ran away from home only to be found sleeping at her father's gravesite. Around that time, Benny came into her life. It is not likely that this girl will ever totally recover. The other daughter, a young teen, met with me. She hated Benny and described unpleasant behaviors like exposing himself, undressing with the bedroom door open and walking in on her while she was in the shower.

The subsequent investigation by Child Protection resulted in Benny's lawyer departing from the case. Benny agreed not to see the children again. Unfortunately, the little girl was too young to give a clear, credible disclosure, so no criminal charges could be pursued. I thought this was the end of it, but I was wrong.

A few months later, Stacia showed up unannounced looking very frightened. She told me that recently her home was broken into and "personal things…only Benny would know about," were stolen. Then this morning, she went into the cellar for something and found all five smoke detectors had been disconnected. They were hard-wired and were disconnected by someone who knew what to do. She said that Benny had threatened to kill all of them and she now feared he would do it. Besides Stacia and her daughters, six children and five adults lived in the building's other apartments. There was a lot to be concerned about.

I immediately called the police and fire departments and the state Fire Marshall's office.

There was no proof that Benny disconnected the smoke detectors, so no charges were ever pursued. However, it appears that Benny was "convinced" that nothing bad better happen in that home or he would be the first suspect. The house was not burned and the harassment stopped.

A year later, I was giving a talk on addiction to a large civic group. There, in the front row was Benny – smiling that Cheshire cat grin throughout my whole presentation. He still owns a lucrative business and generously supports civic organizations. He got away with his crime, and I am convinced that he nearly got away with murder.

Both Philip's mother and Benny hurt those they were supposed to love for no other reason than it made them feel good. They took trust and used it to crush innocence. They found someone easy to manipulate – a drug-dependent family member. My clients were often told that being an addict or an alcoholic is like painting a big target on your back and telling everyone, "Take your best shot…" A truly evil person in each of these cases did just that. They tried to destroy someone who loved and needed them and then justified their actions for their own personal gain. They hurt others simply because it gave them power and control. **This is how you define evil.**

I do not want to bring morality into this book and I do not know if there is a God or a "Higher Power" any more than anyone else does – for why would we need faith if we could prove or disprove the existence of God? I know that the roof creaks when I walk into a church, but that is another story. However, if there is a force of evil, as I felt in these two people, then there must be a force for good. I have witnessed the power of good in the recovery of drug-ravaged lives brought full circle. These are not people who, "got religion" nor are they the ones who talk about their beliefs, for most in recovery keep their faith to themselves. Those who recover use their beliefs as a way to overcome the fears and pain that drove them to use drugs or alcohol in the first place. Terry (page 139) once told me that he was losing all his fears, "because I'm starting to believe in a higher power." I asked what he meant and he explained, "Fear is a lack of faith. If you believe in God, you have to believe he will take care of you. So what is there to be afraid of? I turn everything over to Him each day." Personally, I like that thinking. Nothing preachy. No bible-thumping, and nothing judgmental. For most, spirituality is just an uncomplicated faith that makes recovery easier.

Finally, a thought for those providing treatment or counseling: you will meet wonderfully good people and horribly bad people in this work. Most clients will be burdened by guilt, fear and loneliness. But remember, although they carry labels indicating every personality disorder and mental health problem you can imagine, and a few you cannot, most have lived lives of loss, suffering and abuse that molded them into what they are. Work with each providing guidance and consideration, for you may be the person who saves them.

Summary:

Recovery is hard to define. For most, it is more than just not using drugs. In Twelve-step based recovery programs, the emphasis is on more than physical abstinence. Recovery is elimination of unhealthy and negative behaviors while making changes aimed at self-improvement.

- *Detoxification: provides physical recovery.*
- *Rehabilitation: provides mental, psychological growth via counseling and self-help.*
- *Value or Spiritual Recovery: helps the addict recognize and clarify what led up to their addiction and develop an acceptable set of values to live by.*
- *Chemical Recovery: occurs as drug-free neural responses within the brain change by responding to stress without the need for drugs.*

Most who recover from addiction exhibit some sort of positive change in their value system, either by renewed faith, establishment of improved personal standards or by committing to moral changes in their lives. Belief in God is not necessary for value recovery.

Those who are evil hurt others simply because it gives them power and control. If there is a Power of Evil, there must also be a Power of Good. The power of Good is seen as we witness drug-ravaged lives brought full circle into recovery. The Power of Good does not mean that those in recovery "get religion." It allows them to use their beliefs to overcome the fears and pain that fed into their addictions in the first place.

CHAPTER 8
MAKING RECOVERY WORK

A goal of this book has been to provide the reader with an understanding of not only *addiction* but also of *recovery*. Too often *recovery* is viewed from an "all or nothing" viewpoint – either the person stops all drug and alcohol use immediately on his or her first attempt or that person is a dismal failure and deserves to be abandoned by loved ones and family. No! That is not how it works. Recovery is not a final achievement, it is an ongoing, lifelong process, one often fraught with repeated failures. *Remember, the diseases of addiction are never cured, but their progression can be arrested.*

Like addiction itself, recovery also comes in a lot of different versions. *For that matter, very few will enter a rehabilitation program, counseling or self help and never use again, for relapse is part of the recovery process, especially in early recovery, for most people.* I have known many – not only my clients but friends and associates in self help – who *needed* to relapse in order to find recovery. Almost none get it 100% right the first time, the tenth time or sometimes even at all. For many in the *process of recovery,* if they are making progress by improving their relationships and working toward becoming happier, more confident and content people without drugs or alcohol, they may indeed be achieving recovery, even without total abstinence. For some, sadly, complete abstinence may not be possible. However, if they move toward that goal, they may indeed be achieving recovery, for *recovery is in the process.*

What follows are things that work, and some things that work better than others. Perhaps the worst mistake therapists, doctors, families and those of us who are victims of addiction can make is to try one thing and then give up, viewing the whole process as futile. Although the vignettes in the previous chapters make it appear that treatment is almost always successful, most of my clients over the years tried and failed repeatedly before finally overcoming their addictions. I might also add that I saw as many die trying as I saw succeed. Addiction treatment can be painfully tragic.

Remember, there are many ways to achieve Recovery. Some things work better than others and many in Recovery will use more than one approach to overcoming their addictions. But if something works for you and gives you back your health, self-respect and ability to function as a spouse, parent, employee, friend, citizen or other, then that something is successful – at least for you.

TEN METHODS THAT WORK

1. **Self Help** The most successful approach to recovery, at least as far as anyone can tell, is the *self-help program*. The grand-daddy of self-help, the one upon which most of the other programs are based, is Alcoholics Anonymous. It is the original Twelve Step Program. The *Twelve Suggested Steps* address issues of personal growth centered around: admitting and accepting your addiction; relinquishing attempts to control your addiction by turning it over to others and to a "higher power;" an ongoing process of review of one's character; making amends for harm done by the addiction; and the ongoing development of moral and personal growth.

It should be remembered that the Twelve Steps are the basis for most self-help programs, and all the most successful ones. Many of those attempting recovery remove the word "alcohol" if it is not appropriate, and substitute "addiction" or "emotions" or whatever personal demon they are facing to address their problems. The Twelve Suggested Steps are:

1. We admitted that we were powerless over alcohol – that our lives had become unmanageable.
2. Came to believe that a Power greater than ourselves could restore us to sanity.

3. Made a decision to turn our will and our lives over to the care of God *as we understood Him.*
4. Made a searching and fearless moral inventory of ourselves.
5. Admitted to God, to ourselves, and to another human being the exact nature of our wrongs.
6. Were entirely ready to have God remove all these defects of character.
7. Humbly asked Him to remove our shortcomings.
8. Made a list of all persons we had harmed, and became willing to make amends to them all.
9. Made direct amends to such people whenever possible, except when to do so would injure them or others.
10. Continued to take a personal inventory and when we were wrong promptly admitted it.
11. Sought through prayer and meditation to improve our conscious contact with God, as we understood Him, praying only for knowledge of His will for us and the power to carry that out.
12. Having had a spiritual awakening as the result of these Steps, we tried to carry this message to alcoholics, and to practice these principles in all our affairs.

Remember, the Twelve Steps can be applied to any and all addictions. Just remove the word *alcohol* and substitute another addiction. The main difficulty for many, as mentioned earlier, is the reference to "God," or "Higher Power." This creates difficulties for those who have lost their faith, or perhaps never had any, and are too doubting, depressed or angry to practice any beliefs. In response to this, many substitute the AA program itself, a group, a philosophy, a trusted friend in recovery or even an inanimate object as their personal "Higher Power."

Self-help also has a powerful social aspect, helping those in recovery feel less like they are facing recovery all by themselves. *Remember too, there are many Recovery groups that allow for agnosticism or atheism and use philosophies that are not faith based.*

It is difficult to tell just how successful Twelve Step groups are because most do not take attendance nor do they collect dues nor fees. They have few paid administrative staff and keep no records.

There is no money involved except for purchase of necessary materials like literature and rent and no names are kept. Somehow, the Twelve-Step Recovery program not only survives, but manages to prosper. A.A. is a world-wide entity with millions of members.

A final word about Self-help programs. *They never give up. Unlike families, courts, employers and friends, the self-help program will not abandon you. They will be there when you "...hit bottom," and will provide a blueprint for your recovery – no matter what stage your addiction is at.*

2. **Family interventions:** This method is often the first stop on the road to recovery - an intervention. It is most often a treatment professional who does the intervention, functioning as a guide, walking the addict and concerned others through the intervention process. The spouse, family members, friends and employers are usually the ones who take part in the intervention.

Interventions by their nature tend to be confrontational, with each of the family and friends spelling out, in a non-accusatory manner, how the addict's drug or alcohol use has impacted their lives. The treatment professional elicits feedback from each person present, allowing everyone to speak while addressing obstacles that the addict has used in denial of his addiction.

The treatment professional will plan and rehearse the intervention and arrange for ongoing care such as a detoxification or rehabilitation program. The professional will keep the intervention on topic and may even make arrangements for transportation to programs and follow up for the addict and the family. If there are no treatment professionals available, a person in recovery can attempt to guide the intervention process.

3. **Psychological/Psychiatric Interventions:** Psychiatric and psychological interventions help to determine which problems are drug related and which ones are mental health issues. They can direct the addict toward treatment for underlying mental health and emotional problems. This type of treatment provides behavioral techniques that can make remaining drug-free more successful.

Psychiatry differs from psychology in many ways, but one way is very important. Psychiatrists are medical doctors who can prescribe medication and have admitting privileges to hospitals. Psychologists primarily do talk therapy, often working in conjunction with psychiatrists who handle medication referrals as needed. Talk therapy is also called counseling.

Counselors, psychologists and other mental health professionals are specially trained to provide counseling and educational information to those with addictions. They provide the addict with detailed knowledge of addictions as well as directive counseling to help the addict make decisions about their lifestyles. There can be problems if underlying psychiatric conditions and mental health disorders are overlooked or left untreated.

As pointed out in previous chapters, treating addicts with addictive medications can be difficult. Patients with addictions frequently do not respond well to treatment with addictive drugs. This makes referrals to psychiatrists difficult and explains why successful treatment usually results from psychiatrists and counselors working closely together.

Psychiatry and psychology, along with the educational components of counseling, address many issues related to addiction. Among these are: *Codependence, (def.) the excessive dependence upon a partner who requires much emotional support due to addiction.* The etiology (cause) of addiction and its genetic components can also be clarified, explaining to the addict and family some of the issues that lead to development of the addiction. In addition, factors such as Personality Disorders, dual diagnoses problems (a mix of mental health and drug problems) and family factors ranging from poor communication to domestic violence can be addressed.

4. **Medication:** It is an issue that should always be addressed in treatment and rehabilitation programs. Tragically, many seeking treatment for addiction began their problems with overprescribing from a well-meaning doctor who knew little or nothing about addiction. Medications are often successfully used for relapse prevention, pain management, sleep problems and emotional stability. When treating someone with an addiction however, any previous history of

alcohol or drug use *must* be pursued to ensure that a relapse is not triggered or worse, that the patient is not simply seeking drugs.

Treatment by a physician to address emotional problems like depression or anxiety or debilitating issues like chronic pain are appropriate and effective. Preventative medications such as Disulfiram (Antabuse), to address alcoholism, and antagonist medications like methadone, naltrexone and buprenorphine for opioid addiction can be very effective. The prescribing physician should make himself as familiar as possible with the dangers of over-prescribing as well as his patient's personal history.

It needs to be emphasized that any use of psychotropic (mind-altering) medication for someone with an addiction should be closely monitored by both the counselor and the physician for signs of abuse, which can be either intentional or accidental.

5. **Legal Intervention:** Frequently, it is a personal crisis that forces an alcoholic or drug addict into treatment. One of the most effective ways to create this "moment of truth" for an addict is to get the court involved in the addict's life. Often it is a pending divorce, a DUI (drunk driving) arrest, an assault or something as simple as an arrest for disturbing the peace that forces an addict to seek help. Such a moment often brings the realization that a lawyer is about to enter your life.

It needs to be noted here that no legal action should be taken lightly. Early in my career I was working closely with probation officers who complained that almost all their cases were related to alcohol or drugs. I learned quickly that an incident such as a DUI or a divorce can effectively ruin your life. When all else fails however, an arrest or legal action can jar an addict's life and usually get his attention.

In cases of chronic, late-stage addiction, addicts can be forced into involuntary treatment, usually inpatient care, where hopefully the process of recovery can begin.

6. **Education:** Among the many components of treatment is a strong educational piece to aid in the understanding of

addiction. This is effective because those new to recovery often respond well when they learn about what just kicked the daylights out of their lives. The educational component of a recovery program often provides hope to addicts who, by the time they reach treatment, feel defeated. Education should be provided by a professional, someone knowledgeable about addiction or at least a trusted and successfully sober friend in self-help.

Knowledge does not guarantee anything. It does however, provide an explanation as to why an addict does what he does and can offer strong motivation for recovery. Also, there is a lot of false information out there, so education can help fend off falsehoods that lead to problems. Such information can be found when proponents claim certain drugs are "harmless, non-addictive, safe, do not promote violence and do not affect driving," whether these statements can be proven or not. With many factors affecting addiction, such as the age of the user, the strength of the drug and the mental status of those using a drug, no one attempting to recover from an addiction should use any drug or medication without medical supervision. Failure to discuss the dangers of drug use easily neglects the truth. Early education can address these non-truths and keep those new in recovery from making tragic mistakes.

7. **Rehabilitation Programs:** This is what is usually meant when someone is told they need to "go into treatment." Rehabilitation programs, or "rehab…" can be either inpatient or outpatient, short term or long term and may or may not involve a medical detoxification. These programs come with an inherent problem however: rehabilitation programs, both inpatient and outpatient, often fail to meet expectations by promising too much and delivering too little. They are expensive and can leave an already stressed-out family burdened with a pricey bill for treatment that comes with few guarantees. That being said, a major problem with all drug treatment is that it is impossible to measure success - not only for rehabilitation programs but for any kind of treatment, inpatient or outpatient.

Most inpatient rehab programs have numerous components in common. There is daily group and individual counseling, educational groups and therapy to address all types of issues, both mental and physical, related to the addiction. Many programs offer specialized treatment from acupuncture to family therapy and psychological testing. These programs often work but are most effective when proper *aftercare* is provided. Aftercare means ongoing counseling, support groups and referrals for self-help. *The more follow-up there is, the more success will be seen.*

8. **Faith:** Many who recover, especially those who recover with the aid of self-help programs like AA, find or develop some type of faith. It is usually a simple change, allowing those in recovery to relinquish the need to control everything in their life. Some "find God or Jesus," others find a simple way to pray, yet others develop a personalized faith in a "Higher Power." One of the first people I heard at an A.A. meeting said he started each day by saying, "Hey God, take care of a fool today." At night he looked up and said one word, "Thanks." Whatever works.

The self-help philosophy toward God works for most due to its simplicity. It encourages a simple understanding that it helps a lot if you turn your addiction over to someone or something else. The whole idea is to stop trying to handle your addiction alone, since this has not been working too well up to now. Instead, let go of the need to control what you cannot handle and let help come from elsewhere else.

There is a strong difference between *religion and spirituality. Religion is based upon a belief in God. Spirituality is based upon improving one's moral and ethical values.* It is beliefs put into practice. Those who practice the spirituality found in recovery programs are less concerned with others and more concerned with undoing and avoiding their own mistakes. There is less about judgment and more with self improvement. As said by a very wise client, "The religious are afraid of going to Hell, the spiritual have already been there."

9. **The Power of Example:** It is said that the greatest gift we give others is the power of our own example. This is certainly true when looking at the example we give our children and those around us: spouses, friends and co-workers. They have seen us at our worst when we used drugs seeking unhealthy answers to deadly problems. But in recovery, they see us turn our lives around, becoming what we should be, improving and growing our sense of values.

For those in recovery, remember that even if you relapse, those in your life will see your attempts at recovery and the changes you make. They will see your growth. The power of your example will show others strength and resolve that previously you tried and failed to find through chemicals or unhealthy behaviors.

10. **The Al-Anon Approach:** Al-Anon (and similar groups like Narc-Anon) is a support group for the families and friends of those affected by alcohol and other addictions. Al-Anon was originally developed by spouses of alcoholics who were seeking a support group for themselves. Like A.A., other support groups have spun off Al-Anon and it is now the "grand-daddy" of many similar support groups.

Those closest to the addict often suffer the most. The Al-Anon program is a mutual support group providing suggestions to address the addict's unhealthy behaviors. It is not run by paid professionals but is made up of members who share their "experience, strength and hope" with each other while providing support for the family, not just the addict.

Al-Anon addresses addiction as a family illness. It helps family and friends of addicts stop *enabling* the addict to continue with unhealthy behaviors. It provides strong emotional support for those being affected by someone else's addiction. *It provides specific, practical suggestions for those suffering from a loved one's addiction.*

It is vital to remember, Al-Anon (and programs like it) are highly successful at helping family and friends of addicts change their own behaviors, making them less likely to provide the addict with unhealthy excuses for their addiction.

Summary:

Recovery is not an "all or nothing" pursuit nor is it a lone achievement. It is   an ongoing, lifelong process often with repeated relapses. Addictions are never cured
but their progress can be arrested. Few people recover on their first attempt, for relapse is part of the recovery process.

There are suggested changes that work, and some work better than others. But remember, these are only suggestions. What works for you may not work for others:

1. *Self-Help: By far the most successful approach, most self-help groups are based upon the Twelve Step model and can be applied to all addictions. Self-help does not give up on anyone. It is self-supporting, usually has little or no money involved and no organized leadership. Self-help addresses issues beyond mere physical addiction.*

2. *Family Intervention: Often the first step toward recovery, an intervention is usually done by a treatment professional who walks with the addict, family and friends through a confrontation and referral process. It is designed to force an addict into treatment.*

3. *Psychological/Psychiatric Interventions: These provide referrals to treatment for underlying emotional and mental health issues. They offer behavioral techniques that make staying drug free more successful. Psychiatry can provide medications and hospitalizations. Psychology and counseling are mainly talk therapy. Remember, addicts often do not do well with addictive medications. Talk therapy provides educational components addressing issues like codependency, dual diagnosis issues and family issues like communication and domestic violence.*

4. *Medication: Issues that should always be addressed, over-prescribing and failing to monitor prescriptions can initiate a relapse or an addiction. Maintenance medications can be used for relapse prevention, pain management, sleep problems, depression, anxiety and emotional stability. Also, preventative medications like disulfiram (Antabuse) and antagonist medications like methadone, naltrexone and buprenorphine can be very effective. Any history with drugs or alcohol must be addressed to ensure a relapse is not initiated and all meds must be monitored for signs and symptoms of abuse.*

5. *Legal Intervention: A legal problem can be the "moment of truth" forcing an addict into treatment. However, an arrest can effectively ruin someone's life, so this needs to be approached with caution. Also, late-stage addicts and alcoholics can be forced into treatment in some states.*

6. *Education: Often effective early in treatment, knowledge dispensed by a treatment professional can provide strong motivation for recovery. It fends off falsehoods and misinformation that can lead to trouble.*

7. *Rehabilitation Programs: Often referred to as "going to rehab," they can be either inpatient or outpatient, long-term or short term, with or without a detoxification depending upon medical needs. However, results are often disappointing because much is promised but success cannot be measured. Residential programs are expensive and can be a burden on families. "Aftercare," an ongoing follow-up system of counseling, groups and self-help is vital to the success of rehabilitation programs once they are completed.*

8. *Faith: Many who recover develop some type of faith, whether it was there or not prior to the addiction.*

Discussion of faith often pushes people away since it is a very touchy subject for many in their first approach to recovery, especially those who have lost previous beliefs. So, it should be approached carefully. Development of faith or beliefs can help many overcome feelings of guilt, hopelessness and anger often encountered while new to recovery. This can occur by finding faith in God or through development of a strong sense of values. Some pray, some just turn over their problems to a "higher power" so they do not have to handle things alone. Religion and spirituality differ. Religion is based on a belief in God. Spirituality is based on an improvement in one's values.

9. *Power of Example: It is said that the greatest gift we give others is the power of our own example. Those around an addict see the worst of it when the addiction is at its worst. In recovery, they often see an addict at his best. Even in relapse, there can be a positive effect upon those around the addict as he struggles to recover.*

10. *Al-Anon Approach: Al-Anon and similar programs are support groups for the families and friends of those affected by alcohol or drugs. It was developed as a support for spouses only but now is for anyone concerned. Those closest to an addict suffer the most. Al-Anon, Narc-Anon and similar groups provide support and advice to help overcome the addict's behaviors. It helps stop "enabling" behaviors and provides specific suggestions for those suffering from a loved one's addiction.*

CHAPTER 9
TRANSITIONS

By 1998, I was comfortably ensconced in the methadone clinic. It was a lot like having an independent practice, except that I worked under the clinic's license rather than my own. I ran groups, saw a large caseload and felt that overall, I had found my place. The clients were fascinating and challenging and some actually achieved recovery. I looked forward to going to work daily, which is more than a lot of people can say. I had it made. But one night, my life changed.

My wife was chronically ill with diabetes and a litany of related physical and psychological ills. She was also a smoker. Try as she might with nicotine-laced gum, pills, therapists and even a hypnotist, she kept returning to cigarettes. She developed lung disease and was on breathing medications and machines to keep her lungs open. One Friday night her smoking triggered an asthma attack. She stopped breathing and went into cardiac arrest before my eyes. She died two weeks later, having never regained consciousness. The irony cannot be missed. I spent my life treating addictions, only to have my wife die from one before my eyes. Donna was forty-six.

There is no way to prepare for a loved-one's death. No matter how hard we try or how sure we are that everything will be managed, it is still hard as hell to endure. Donna's death left me with a grieving nine-year-old son and sixteen-year-old daughter. I quickly learned the difficulties of being a single parent. About a week after my children returned to school following Donna's death, her best friend showed up in the afternoon to watch over my son. She found him sitting at our computer logged onto a program allowing him to send an E-mail to Heaven. He was all alone, writing a letter to Mom, tears streaming down his cheeks. That day, I made a decision to change my career.

Addicts die. More accurately, they die young. The average alcoholic lives twelve years less than the general population. When combined with the effects of cigarettes, the chances of an alcoholic dying from throat cancer is multiplied by a factor of fifty. The cardio-pulmonary damage from nicotine is well documented, leaving its victims debilitated and the quality of life diminished. Heroin and cocaine addicts drop quickly from both the powerful physical damage inflicted by drugs and through the overall lifestyle which often brings with it dangerous circumstances and companions. It is said in A.A. that there are a lot of old drunks around but almost no old addicts. However, the most widely used drug is still nicotine, killing over 100,000 Americans each year. I doubt Donna ever thought that middle age for her would be 23 years old.

Addiction treatment requires a lot of dedication. Group therapies are usually held in the evening when the maximum number of clients is available. Individual sessions are scheduled around times before clients go to work or later when they are returning. This required a lot of hours in the office. There were years of early morning meetings and missed dinners. No more. Now I had to be home for my children.

I initially brought my decision to leave to one of my therapy groups. It was made up mostly of "old timers," addicts who had been in recovery for more than a year and were rebuilding their lives. One woman in the group said it best. "What good is your life if your kids get all screwed up because you work too many hours? You always want us to do the right thing. Now you need to do the right thing. You need to be home for your kids." I submitted my resignation that week.

When I told my colleagues of my decision to leave, some hugged me, others shook my hand. They took me to lunch and parceled out my caseload. When I told my clients of my decision, many of them cried. I was hugged and thanked. Jorge, a warm, sensitive Hispanic man shared the death of his own wife and the decisions he was forced to make. We both cried as we compared our pain. Two of my clients opened up about the deaths of children, pain they had kept locked away for fear of reopening wounds they could not handle. Many of my clients had HIV and were themselves facing death. Now they talked more openly, with more than one asking, "I wonder if anyone will miss me when I'm gone." Death once again put a new perspective on life.

The week before I left, I received a phone call from the roommate of my next appointment, Jimmy. The roommate just got a call telling him that Jimmy's mother had died suddenly. I had to break the news to Jimmy. It was a long meeting that day. Jimmy, dying from HIV himself, talked about his mother and his regrets over the pain he caused her. He told me he recently reconciled with his family, including his mother, and said this was the only thing he had done right in the past few years. He smiled about that. "At least Mom died knowing I'm not using any more." That is one way of measuring success.

A few weeks after Donna's death, I went to work for the Department of Children and Families, (DCF) the state agency given the job of protecting children from child abuse and neglect. Still, I found myself working with addictions. According to The Department of Health and Human Services, at least three of every five cases of child abuse and endangerment are related to problems with alcohol and drugs. Abuse cases are often the most spectacular. There are those who are mentally ill and those who are sexual perverts and those who are just mean and abusive. But for the most part, abuse comes from drunk or addicted parents who can barely take care of themselves, let alone their children. Acts of abuse are often committed by parents who grew up the same way – for child abuse is generational, just like addiction. It is all many of these parents knew and saw while growing up. They often do not even know it is wrong to abuse their children.

Neglect, however, is worse. Neglectful parents are those who let their children grow up in a war zone, witnessing domestic violence, or those who are too wrapped up in their own drug or alcohol use to properly care for their kids. Abusive parents can love their children but not know how to parent properly. Neglectful parents are worse. They send the message that they just do not care. It is their children who most often fall into their own drug dependence or alcoholism at an early age. These are children who grow up *parentified*, caring for their younger siblings or for their own parents who are too debilitated by their addictions to function. These are the children with a distorted self-image, never good enough, always blamed for things that go wrong.

At the Department of Children and Families, the clients are called "consumers." The label has again changed. Yet once again, I find myself staring into the eyes of children who were abused or neglected. I see the reflection of future Reynolds or Terrys. I see those who cannot bond with anyone, and those who have learned to use violence to resolve issues. I see those who have learned only to escape through chemicals. In spite of this, I also see the children who will make it – those who will bond with a healthy person, a family member, perhaps a teacher, a social worker or even a counselor – *perhaps with you.* I see the children who will grow beyond their environments to become productive, healthy and successful. For I see those who will enter the realm of recovery.

I finish with that closing thought. *Recovery.* It is as misunderstood as addiction itself, yet remains the primary goal of addicts and treatment professionals alike. There are many kinds of recovery. Sometime, it occurs even though total abstinence remains elusive. Conversely, there are many who quit drinking or drug use but make no other changes. Talk to their families and you hear things like, "He's more miserable now than when he was getting high." That is not recovery either.

Those who work in the field of addiction treatment will not remain for the money, for it is just not there. It will not be for the praise, nor for the thanks, for those are rare commodities. But they may remain in the field for love. Yeh, that sounds corny as hell. Love. But those treating addictions will be witness to people overcoming abuse that most of us cannot begin to imagine. They will see men and women change in ways deemed impossible by medical experts, psychiatrists and men of God. They will see prostitutes and thieves, killers and con men, the abused and the abusers turn lives around to become successful and generous, and some of the happiest, most grateful people they will ever meet. They will learn that there is indeed nothing like getting knocked on your ass to turn you into a better person. For they will witness the most remarkable turnabout a person can experience. They will witness *recovery.*

CONCLUSION

Very little remains the same since I began as an entry-level counselor in the mid-1970's. Back then, heroin was mainly consigned to inner-cities - today it destroys entire communities, and in many rural as well as urban areas is the #1 cause of death among young adults. Cocaine was pretty much of an unknown entity, found mainly in South American jungles or medical research labs. Today, cocaine has decimated neighborhoods in many cities as drug cartels have spread their tentacles throughout the world via the rich U.S. market. Methamphetamines were unknown to most of law enforcement and the medical community in 1970. Now, they have produced a nightmare of crime and violence throughout the nation. Fentanyl, developed as a powerful pain killer for the terminally ill and those undergoing invasive surgery, has become a societal horror as users of this drug die quickly and often far too young from its incredibly toxic effects. Non-medical marijuana sales (no one called it recreational) used to get people incarcerated for years, but now it is seen as a panacea for states hoping to fill their coffers with easy money. It is now the #1 drug used in America, with 17.7 million using marijuana daily as opposed to 14.7 million who drink alcohol daily. Approximately 40% of marijuana users are using it regularly and it is likely soon to be reclassified as a less dangerous drug. Oh yes, let us not forget alcohol and nicotine, still killing thousands of Americans each year.

Addicts used to be found in inner-city ghettos and addiction was something to be whispered about. In 1970, addictive behavior was dismissed as part of a criminal element or was at most acceptable among edgy populations like musicians. HIV did not yet exist. Today, opioid addiction has damaged the lives of millions of an entire generation after big pharma pursued profits while pretending opiates could be controlled.

Treatment has also changed as improved standards of care developed. No more are insurance companies paying for expensive treatment over and over, but no more are they able to refuse treatment without justification. Treatment itself has improved with better education and mental health services and the advent of improved medications. Aftercare has moved beyond simply sending a client out the door with a phone number for an Alcoholics or

Narcotics Anonymous member. Medical follow-up is markedly better with more focus on addressing a patient's physical, emotional, family and psychiatric needs. Things are better, but there will always be a long way to go.

***

As I completed this book, I read yet another claim that all addictions are some type of mental health disorder. This one stated that all addictions result from painful child trauma and are simply behavioral disorders related to depression. Although childhood trauma is frequently found, it is not the sole causative factor in the development of an addiction. The author, a respected psychiatrist, fails to consider the roles of cultural beliefs, social pressures, physical dependence, age at initial use, peer influence and a litany of other physical, familial and mental health factors that impact the development of an addiction.

Another mental health researcher denies that addictions are diseases and claims they are either the result of maladaptive coping with childhood or some type of severe trauma. Such theories ignore addiction's multitude of causative factors, not the least of which is the powerful, addictive potential of drugs like opiates, crack cocaine, amphetamines, fentanyl and other well-recognized drugs of abuse that create both powerful physical dependence and painful withdrawal *almost overnight*.

Many an addict began their journey by "experimentation" as an adolescent. Many others use addictive drugs to escape emotional issues like divorce, job or financial losses, grief, heartbreak or an anxiety or depressive disorder. Others simply "followed the crowd," starting with what seemed like harmless fun, but soon became hooked on something they never dreamed could destroy their lives. And let us not forget the millions who became addicted due to chronic pain. This does not include the hundreds of thousands who die yearly as a result of nicotine. Many addicts indeed come from horribly abusive and dysfunctional families, but to state that this is the sole reason for the development of addictions is nonsense.

Finally, there is a claim that addictions are a type of obsessive-compulsive disorder. Although characterized by behaviors that are repetitive, destructive and out-of-control, OCD is not the same as the chemically induced behaviors of addiction producing physical withdrawal, compulsive use, binge behavior and physiological damage over time. That physiological damage includes long-term changes in the structure and function of the brain. These changes are caused by addiction – and these changes are, by definition, a disease:

A disease, is defined as, "a condition of abnormal vital function involving any structure, part, or system of an organism…a specific illness or disorder characterized by a recognizable set of signs and symptoms, attributable to heredity, infection, diet or environment." An addiction is far more than a set of behaviors and must be attributed to more than just a change in one's endorphin levels. It is a condition affecting the brain's functioning, caused by factors including family, genetics, social pressures, biochemical and environmental changes and exposure to unhealthy behaviors. These are only some of the many causal factors that create an addiction. Were it simply a set of out-of-control behaviors, an addiction could be easily cured by behavior modification. To deny that addictions are diseases is to deny all the evidence.

***

As I end this book, I realize that not only has change occurred in drug use and treatment, it has also occurred in me. It took me over ten years to write this book, but I realized as I reached my final chapter that addiction can still be diagnosed and understood using one phrase – **"a pattern of problems."** *If your use of a chemical of any kind, either singly or combined with others, causes a pattern of problems that are physical, mental, emotional, social, relational or other and are initiated directly by your use of that chemical, then you are an addict. It really is just that simple.* Many mental health issues like depression, anxiety, OCD or a history of childhood abuse cause problems, terrible problems. However, if they are induced by regular use of a chemical, no matter what other factors exist, they are addictions.

I also reached the understanding that an addict who dies has not wasted his life, he is simply, and tragically, a victim of the terrible disease of addiction. Perhaps this is why the medical, psychiatric, legal and educational professions have so much difficulty defining addiction. The definitions just too simple for experts who have devoted their lives to fighting various aspects of addiction or mental health disorders.

It is also not for the addict to self-diagnose, for addiction is called the "disease of denial" for a reason. Those of us who provide treatment have seen dozens go to their grave denying that their drug use was a problem. So, we should all keep in mind that if anyone in your life dislikes something about your behavior because of your drug or alcohol use, consider yourself diagnosed.

How has this happened? *The neuronal structure of your brain has been changed by the use of a drug–and that change is addiction.* The regular use of an addictive substance causes neuronal changes creating an increasingly powerful craving to use. This craving is usually very subtle – so subtle that the brain cannot sense the change until it has already occurred.

I am far less judgmental about those with addictions than I was fifty years ago and now understand how good people fall victim to such a tragic illness as addiction. Is there an easy answer for someone who has become addicted? No. But if you or someone you love is having problems with drugs or alcohol, *seek help and do not stop trying.* The greatest gifts you have to give are your efforts, your love and the power of your own example, for they can indeed save lives.

AFTERWORD

Many people and organizations were vital resources for compilation of the facts within this book. Without the expertise provided to me over the past years by gifted colleagues, friends and supervisors, completion of this text could never have been accomplished. Neither would I have experienced a career that gave me so many opportunities to help those in need. Time has been a harsh teacher however, as many have now passed on and others are faded from my memory, nameless but identifiable to me only through incidents, some poignant, others painful, but all instructive.

I wish to thank the staff of AdCare Hospital (formerly Doctors Hospital of Worcester), where my career began. I also thank Reliant Medical Group (formerly Fallon Clinic), HMA Behavioral Health, Inc., Spectrum Health Services, Inc., Framingham University, University of Massachusetts Medical Center, the Massachusetts Department of Children and Families, the New Beginnings Wellness Center of Worcester, and all others who contributed to a wonderful and sometime wild career in the treatment of addictions. Finally, I must thank the many who years ago welcomed me through the doors of Alcoholics Anonymous. Without their help and support I could not have found in sobriety such a rewarding career.

I also wish to acknowledge the information gleaned from the pages of the *Diagnostic and Statistical Manual of Mental Disorders (DSM V)*, *Mosby's Medical, Nursing and Allied Health Dictionary, 4th ed.*, and *Tabor's Cyclopedic Medical Dictionary, FA Davis Co, 15th edition*.

Without the assistance of the above resources, I could not have completed this text.

Above all, I wish to thank the thousands of clients who passed through my offices. I will be forever grateful for the honesty and pain shared with me over the years. My memories are sometimes clouded by time, but just as often by tears as I recall with warmth my experiences with some of the finest people I ever met. May God bless all of you.

GLOSSARY
OF
ADDICTION TERMINOLOGY

ACUTE:
Sharp or severe. (See Addiction, Stages of)

ACUTE ABSTINENCE SYNDROME:
Withdrawal symptoms, including physical and psychologic, experienced by a chemically dependent person who is suddenly deprived of a regular intake of their drug of choice.

ADDICT:
A person who has become physiologically or psychologically dependent upon a chemical (drugs, alcohol) so that normal social, occupational or other responsible life functions are disrupted. One who is physically or psychologically dependent upon a substance, especially drugs or alcohol, with use of increasing amounts to achieve the desired effect. Also included are gambling and computer addictions, which, although there is no actual chemical dependency, create behaviors identical to chemical addictions without drug involvement.

ADDICTION:
Regularly performed attempts at pleasurable stimulation resulting in a progressive pattern of use, often with mild to extreme craving upon cessation of use. (It features) compulsive, uncontrolled dependence on a substance, habit or practice to such a degree that cessation causes severe emotional, mental or psychologic reactions. The behaviors of addiction are repetitive but not ritualistic.
Note: addiction has multiple definitions usually applicable to the discipline defining it.

ADDICTION, STAGES of: (levels of impairment)

There are three stages of addiction: Early, Acute, Chronic

Early: also called prodromal, pertaining to the early symptoms that may mark the onset of the disease of addiction. *Example*: a pattern of obsession becomes evident as the use of a drug becomes increasingly important in social, emotional or other areas of life.

Acute: Sharp or severe. Having rapid onset, severe symptoms, short course. *Example*: a pattern of problems develops such as using more of a drug than one intended to; social or familial problems related to drug use.

Chronic: Long, drawn out, of long duration. *Example*: A pattern of problems indicating a disease which show little change or slow progression. With addictions, there are usually physical problems from the drug use evident at this point.

The Stages of Addiction are also called *Levels of Impairment.*

ALCOHOLICS ANONYMOUS:

An international, non-profit organization consisting of abstinent alcoholics and/or drug addicts whose sole purpose is to stay sober and help each other to achieve sobriety. It works through group support, shared experiences, and faith in a "higher power, if so desired" while avoiding allegiance to any specific religion or sect. Philosophical practice is to live "one day at a time." The only desire for membership is the desire to stop drinking. Among program spinoffs are Narcotics Anonymous, Al-Anon, Alateen, all of which offer support. It is highly successful as a support for those in recovery and can be used as an adjunct to other programs.

CANNABIS:

Cannabis sativa is the common hemp plant from which cannabis is obtained. All parts of the plant contain cannabinoids, the psychoactive substances in the plant. THC (tetrahydrocannabinol) is the isomer that is believed to cause the characteristic psychologic effects including alterations of mood, memory, motor coordination, cognitive ability, and self-perception. Cannabis use has been decriminalized in many states and recreational use is legalized in others. There are multiple medicinal uses for cannabis, which can be ingested orally, via capsule, smoked or dermally among other methods. Excessive use of cannabis can cause cannabism, characterized by anxiety, disorientation, hallucinations, memory defects and paranoia. Long term use is linked to cannabinoid emesis disorder.

CHEMICAL DEPENDENCE:

The total psychophysical state of one addicted to drugs or alcohol who must receive an increasing amount of the substance to prevent the onset of abstinence symptoms. Commonly called addiction.

CHEMICAL RECOVERY:

Change that occurs within the brain affecting neural responses to stressors like pain, fear, anxiety and anger. With chemical Recovery, the body develops internal strengths that do not require the use of drugs to address the stressors. Confidence increases as skills and maturity grow and the values become clarified.

COCAINE HYDROCHLORIDE:

Cocaine hydrochloride is a white crystalline powder originally used as a topical anesthetic. It is derived from the cocoa plant but is also prepared synthetically. It has a high potential for addiction. Cocaine is used as a local analgesic however it is highly toxic with serious psychotropic effects. Symptoms include nervous excitement, restlessness, incoherent speech, fever, hypertension, cardiac arrythmias, convulsions, respiratory arrest and death. (see crack cocaine)

COMPULSION:

Very noticeable in the chronic or late stage of addiction, compulsion is characterized by binge or out-of-control drug or alcohol use that is easily triggered. It occurs when physical contact with a drug is again made after a period or time or an attempt to stop using. It is often contrary to one's ordinary judgements or standards and is triggered by or the result of obsession. (see obsession)

CRACK COCAINE:

A smokeable form of cocaine, it is small pieces of cocaine hydrochloride base chemically separated from its impurities. It is cracked into small pieces to be smoked, hence the name "crack." Highly addictive, users can exhibit withdrawal and compulsive use rapidly, often within weeks or even days of initial use. Smoking cocaine is also called "freebasing."

CROSS ADDICTION:

The understanding that if you are addicted to a drug, you are addicted to all drugs of the same family. For example, if addicted to one amphetamine, you are addicted to all amphetamines. If addicted to a sedative hypnotic, you are addicted to all sedative hypnotics. If a heroin or other opioid addict uses alcohol, he is extremely high risk to develop alcoholism, since both are sedatives. (see cross tolerance)

CROSS TOLERANCE:

A tolerance to other drugs of the same type or family that develops after exposure to only one agent. An example is the cross tolerance that develops between alcohol and barbiturates. (see cross addiction)

DETOXIFICATION:

Detoxification or "detox" is the medical process of removing the physiological effects of alcohol and/or drugs which have been smoked, snorted, injected, eaten, inhaled or otherwise ingested from a patient's system while minimizing serious withdrawal or side effects.

DISEASE OF ADDICTION:

A disease is a condition of abnormal vital functioning involving any structure, part or system of an organism…a specific illness or disorder characterized by recognizable signs and symptoms attributable to heredity, infection, disease or environment. The disease of addiction is out-of-control physical and/or psychological dependence on a substance, esp. drugs or alcohol, with use of increasing amounts. All addictions have three stages: early (prodromal), acute (severe), chronic (long term, noncommunicable).

FENTANYL CITRATE:
A potent synthetic narcotic analgesic. The trade name is sublimaze. It is used primarily as an adjunct to general preoperative and postoperative anesthesia. It is highly addictive and extremely toxic and is responsible for many overdose deaths. It is commonly used as a cut for heroin or other illicit drugs of abuse.

GAMBLING ADDICTION:
Viewed as a psychological problem, often as a form of Obsessive-Compulsive-Disorder, gambling has the behavioral and psychological characteristics of a chemical addiction. These characteristics (Obsession, Compulsion and Progression, Relapse) are as evident with a gambler as with a relapsing drug addict. However, the difference is that drug addiction always has a chemical component, whereas a gambling addiction is behavioral, with no chemical involvement.

Note: excessive computer use is also considered by some to be an addiction although it is not, as of this writing, classified as a psychiatric or mental health disorder or addictive disorder. Like gambling, it has the characteristics of an addiction but without a chemical component.

HABITUATION:
Psychological or emotional dependence upon a drug, tobacco or alcohol resulting from repeated use of the substance but without the addictive, physiologic need to increase dosage.

The act of becoming accustomed to anything from frequent usage. In addiction the mental equivalent of physical tolerance and dependence on drugs.

HIV (Human Immunodeficiency Virus)
HIV is the retrovirus that causes AIDS. It is transmitted through contact with an infected individual's blood, semen, cervical secretions, cerebrospinal fluid or synovial fluid. HIV infects the T-cells of the immune system and results in an infection with an incubation period of up to ten years. With the immune system destroyed, AIDS develops as opportunistic infections and attacks organ systems throughout the body. Among intravenous drug users,

the virus is spread easily by sharing bodily fluids through the use of needles and exposure through sexual contact.

METHADONE HYDROCHLORIDE:

A synthetic narcotic analgesic used primarily as a substitute for heroin, allowing withdrawal without development of acute abstinence syndrome. Methadone is used primarily for detoxification from opioids or in the treatment of opioid addiction. It is used for pain relief under the label Dolophine.

METHADONE MAINTENANCE:

A daily or regular therapeutic dosage of methadone that keeps withdrawal symptoms away while blocking the effects of other opioids like heroin or opioid medications. It is low cost, covered by many third-party payers and is used for long-term opioid addiction treatment. It is found to be more successful the longer patients remain in treatment.

METHAMPHETAMINE:

Methamphetamine is a synthetic amphetamine, a form of speed, that is ingested in similar ways to cocaine. Longer lasting than cocaine, users can stay "high" for 4-5 days with violent and paranoid symptoms. Extreme potential for addiction.

OBSESSION:

(1) The mental state of having an uncontrollable desire to dwell on an idea or an emotion.

(2) A persistent, repetitive thought involving the use of alcohol, drugs or their related behaviors with which the mind is regularly preoccupied and suggests an act requiring the use of these substances. It is the first factor found in the development of an addiction: (obsession, compulsion, progression, relapse.)

(3) Obsession is the preoccupation with one's drug of choice and the related behaviors which leads to continued use despite other intentions. (see compulsion)

OBSESSIVE-COMPULSIVE DISORDER:

Obsessive-compulsive disorder is characterized by the presence of obsessions, which are recurrent and persistent thoughts, urges, or images that are experienced as intrusive and unwanted. Obsessive-Compulsive Behaviors commonly accompany these compulsions. These are repetitive behaviors or mental acts that an individual feels driven to perform in response to an obsession or according to rules that must be applied rigidly. Addictions can be mislabeled as forms of OCD; however, there is little or only incidental chemical involvement with OCD, whereas addictions must have chemical involvement to trigger their repetitive, self-destructive behaviors. Also, obsessions are viewed as ritualistic behaviors, addictions are repetitive behaviors, not ritualistic. (see obsession, compulsion)

OPIATE and OPIOID DEFINITIONS:

An opiate is derived from the opium poppy.

An opioid is any narcotic drug, natural or synthetic, with opium like affects, not necessarily derived from the opium poppy.

PERSONALITY DISORDERS:

An enduring pattern of inner experience and behavior that deviates markedly from the expectations of the individual's culture, is pervasive and inflexible and has an onset in adolescence or early adulthood, is stable over time, and leads to distress or impairment. Personality Disorders are grouped into three clusters based upon similarities. In Cluster B., which includes *Antisocial, Borderline, Histrionic* and *Narcissistic personality disorders*, a high percentage of those with addictions are found.

POST-ACUTE WITHDRAWAL SYNDROME:

Post-acute withdrawal is a long-term condition experienced by many who quit drug and alcohol use. It leaves its victims moody and suffering from insomnia long after they have stopped using.

PROGRESSION:

Term used to describe the course of addiction in which the characteristic signs and symptoms become more prominent and severe over time. It is one of the four characteristics of an addiction: (obsession, compulsion, progression, relapse.)

RECOVERY:

In treatment and self-help programs, the term *recovery* refers to more than abstinence. It is beyond simply physical recovery from an addiction. *Recovery* is the elimination of negative or unhealthy behaviors that lead up to substance use while making changes aimed at self-improvement. It is the process or act of becoming well or returning to a state of health through the elimination of drugs and/or alcohol *as well as* elimination of the behaviors that lead up to their use.

Abstinence is viewed as part of recovery, which is an ongoing process. Few who attempt to recover from an addiction will never use again, for relapse, especially early in recovery, is part of the recovery process for most. In self-help programs, recovery is in the process as one continues to make self-improvement over time.

RELAPSE:

Relapse is the recurrence of a disease or symptom after a period of time in recovery. With addictions, relapse is common, especially early in recovery. It is one of the four factors in the development of the disease of addiction. (obsession, compulsion, progression, relapse).

SEDATIVE-HYPNOTIC:

A drug that reversibly depresses the activity of the central nervous system, used to induce sleep and allay anxiety. (Included are) barbiturates and many other non-barbiturate tranquilizers. Drugs in this group have a high potential for abuse that often results in physical and psychologic dependence; treatment of dependence involves gradual reduction of dosage since abrupt withdrawal frequently causes serious disorders, including seizures.

TETRAHYDROCANNABINOL (THC)

Tetrahydrocannabinol is the primary cannabinoid found in marijuana. It is the principal psychoactive substance of cannabis. It is commonly called the delta-9 THC isomer, the primary psychoactive compound in cannabis.

TOLERANCE:

Tolerance is seen when there is a marked increase in the dose of the substance to achieve the desired effect or a markedly reduced effect when the usual dose is consumed. Prime examples are found with the use of opioids. Opioid users will exhibit an increased need to use more of their drug of choice over a period of time as their use continues. Example: Over time, heroin users will use an amount of the drug that would kill a novice user just to fend off withdrawal discomfort. Tolerance varies greatly with an individual's, age, physical size, use of other drugs, overall physical health, length of time using the drug, and the type and strength of drug being used.

TRIGGERS:

A trigger is a substance, object or agent that initiates or stimulates drug use. Also called "cues," triggers often set people on the road to a relapse.

VALUE or SPIRITUAL RECOVERY:

Value or spiritual recovery is recognizing, clarifying and attempting to live up to a culturally acceptable set of standards. The improvements in the value system of the one seeking recovery come after that person has begun to recovery physically and mentally and has made a commitment to facilitate changes to remain drug and alcohol free.

WITHDRAWAL SYNDROME (ACUTE):

A physical reaction after cessation or severe reduction in intake of a substance such as alcohol, opiates or other drugs that have been regularly used to induce euphoria, intoxication or relief from pain or distress. The body tissues become dependent upon the regular reinforcing effect of the chemical so that interruption of the dosage induces an organic mental state characterized by anxiety, insomnia, restlessness, irritability, impaired attention and often physical illness.

www.ingramcontent.com/pod-product-compliance
Lightning Source LLC
LaVergne TN
LVHW052021080426
835513LV00018B/2108